Chapter Four: Empowering And Opening Our Chakras To Improve Ourselves

Chapter Five: Proven Benefits Of Chakra

Conclusion

Crystals For Beginners

Introduction

Many people in the Western World are ignorant of what the chakras are and how they affect our daily lives, including our health! The exciting thing about the chakras is that, like gravity, whether or not you pay attention to them, they play a role in your emotional, physical, and spiritual health. Even if you're new to researching holistic wellbeing and complementary medicine, or even other philosophical concepts and theosophical practices, getting a good understanding of this complex energy network would certainly help everyone.

In this book, we're going to discuss how energy healing helps balance the seven main chakras. It's very typical in today's world, with busy schedules, unhealthy diets and lack of sleep, to find our chakras unbalanced. I'd say most people don't even know how to control their chakras. But this book, I would hope they do. Energy healing is going to allow you to get back in touch with your body. Chakra energy healing will also help you feel balanced, complete, and influences your overall well- being. There are quite a number of different ways to perform chakra healing. Ensure that the energy healing technique of the chakra sounds right for you and that you're confident with it.

Chakra meditation is a great way to improve your spiritual wellbeing and health. You shift your energy by meditating on the chakra. Not only do you feel better when you change your attitude, but it can also help you move more quickly along your path. That's why meditation on the chakra can be great if you feel blocked in any way. Keeping your energy clean and flowing allows you to connect to a higher degree of vibration. Your Self and the Cosmos (God, Higher Source, etc.) interact more easily because the World does not have to go through all the energy muck that is stored in your energy system.

What you're going to get from this book is understanding how to achieve a healed and balanced chakra system. Once equilibrium is reached, absolutely everything works at its best. Our environment, our bodies, our strength, our government, the World, the tides, the atmosphere, the water cycle, and all other spheres within our life need to be balanced to function fully. A well-balanced body starts with a well-balanced diet, a well-balanced environment, and an understanding of the need to balance the seven chakras.

Well, there are proven benefits of knowing the chakras and how we can improve ourselves by opening and accessing the energy of each of our magic chakras, all of which are discussed in this book. So, without further delay, let's go straight to it, and you'll be astounded by the power that each chakra can offer to your life.

CHAPTER ONE

What Are Chakras?

C hakras are simply energy centers inside the body. This ancient Sanskrit term translates as "the wheels of fire." These light wheels are located vertically in the center of your body, approximately aligned with your spine. Each chakra affects and reflects a particular area of the body. As you learn how each one affects your wellbeing, you can also learn how to enhance the quality of your overall condition by opening, clearing, improving, and recognizing your chakras.

Chakras can be explained as places in our body where the universal life-force (kundalini) is particularly concentrated and leads to tangible experiences at the physical, emotional and spiritual levels. Everyone has life-force/kundalini energy to some degree – so, in everyone, the chakras are active to some degree and can be felt-either in a pleasurable way or in a distorted and painful way.

In various cultures of the world, there are multiple structures and hypotheses about the various chakras and energy channels in the human body. For example, the Hindu system recognizes seven key chakras, while the Tibetan Buddhist system has only five. Yet the other systems describe three, nine or even 12 key chakras.

What is important to understand is that chakras and energy channels are not a mechanical system of pipes and vents in our body through which energy flows, but are highly individual experiences at the physical, emotional and spiritual levels. In other words, there are very different perceptions of the chakras in our bodies.

Scientists and researchers at Jiao Tong University in Shanghai, using advanced and powerful scientific instruments, have shown that subtle energy has the characteristics of electromagnetic current when flowing through acupuncture meridians, but that it has the properties of coherent particle streams, similar to laser light when projected out of the body by master

Qigong healers who cure diseases. Some understanding of the mechanism and dynamics of the chakras would help us to understand how we can beam the energy (which is manifested as a coherent light) from the chakras.

How are Chakras formed?

Barbara Brennan, a former NASA engineer and now a world- renowned energy healer, describes chakras as "swirling cone- shaped vortexes in the field of human energy." From this perspective, chakras, plasma metaphysics (or "wheels" in Sanskrit) can be considered to be made up of two components: one, a magnetized node and two, a rotating cone structure or a vortex that forms in low-density magnetic plasma.

Recent laboratory experiments have shown that a regional source at a fixed frequency stimulates a cone of cosmic ray in a plasma crystal. The apex of the circles will be pointed to the source and the angle of the cone will be determined by the frequency of the spin. Excitations from fast-moving particles in a plane below or near a single-layer plasma crystal give rise to these cones. According to plasma cosmology, when filamentary currents pinch, rotating galaxies in space are formed. This can happen when two currents pass toward or cross each other. Dr. David Tansely, a radionics specialist, says, "Seven main chakras are established at points where standing lines of lights (or meridians) cross each other 21 times. The 21 minor chakras are situated at points where energy strands cross 14 times." On the basis of these theories, we can infer how chakras develop in subtle bodies (composed of magnetic plasma or "magma").

When the meridians cross our subtle bodies, they pinch each other, forming "knots" and collapsing like dense nodes of strong magnetic fields pulsating at fixed frequencies. Super particles and objects are drawn to magnetized nodes and drawn into subtle bodies at very high speeds using helical paths. This dynamic nature of the incoming particles and the pulsation of the node stimulates the cone structures on the surface of the body. Plasma of charged particles (popularly known in philosophical literature as "qi," "prana" or "kundalini"), from the ionized world, spirals to the nodes, spinning the magnetic plasma on the surface of the small, subtle body. It is often absorbed into the chakra, and its energy is then transferred to the various parts of the subtle body through a network of meridians (or filamentary currents) within the body.

Chakra Structure

According to scientific researchers, the dynamic elastic double vortex structure emanates from the excited region of the plasma crystal. Each region is divided into an outgoing and inward-looking vortex. The wave-fronts are circular in the vicinity of the source. This is close to how theoretical metaphysicists, such as Charles Leadbeater and Brennan, described and demonstrated the spinal chakras – which come in pairs and have circular wave-fronts. The tube or channel connects the outward-facing chakra at the front of the body to the chakra behind the body, which faces in the opposite direction.

According to scientific researchers, plasma crystal cones have an unusual multiple structure of nested cones. Brennan found evidence of the nested cones within the chakras in our magnetic plasma bodies. According to Brennan, the chakras appear "to be nestled within each other like nesting glasses. Each chakra on each higher layer extends further into the auric field (to the edge of each auric layer) and is slightly wider than the one below it." Each vortex metabolizes the energy that resonates with its specific spin frequency.

Alignment of Chakras

It is important to note that the cone structures of the chakras in metaphysical literature are located in various angles. As noted above, the angle corresponds to the frequency of the radiation source. It is well known in metaphysics that not only are the spinal chakras located at different angles, but each chakra spins at a different frequency. The axis of each cone is connected with the magnetic field generated by the node so that the cone apex of the chakra facing the central channels of the subtle body has a various magnetic polarity from the base of the cone. When we consider the central channel in the subtle body, the nodes in the central channels would be distributed discreetly. This is consistent with metaphysical observations (and is consistent with the behavior of magnetic plasma observed in plasma crystal studies). According to

Brennan, "Their tips point to the main vertical current and their open ends extend to the edges of each layer of the field in which they are located."

Absorption and Emission of Chakra Energy

Brennan stated that every whirling vortex of energy appears to be sucking or energizing energy from the universal energy field. Chakras are related to meridian points, which are regions with strong magnetic fields. They are therefore capable of attracting super-particles and objects charged with high energy. Particles, after absorption, run through the meridians to distribute energy to different parts of the body – similar to what occurs in the heart-lung and circulatory systems in the physico-biomolecular body in terms of the distribution of oxygen to the cells in the body. When the particles in the subtle bodies are energized, they begin to respond to their environment. Leadbeater states that one of the functions of the chakras is to calibrate (or input) the frequency of the particles in order to respond to particular radiation frequencies in the environment. Brennan also points out that the direction in which the chakra spins is significant. When the chakra spins clockwise, it absorbs energy. When spinning in the opposite direction, the flow of energy is in the inverted direction. In other words, it emits energy rather than absorbs it.

Focused Light Beams from Rotating Galaxies

According to scientific researchers, the ordered magnetic field plays a key role in the formation of jets from a rotating accretion disk in an ionized environment. The process of forming jets (or focused light beams) is thought to depend on how magnetic fields act when they are swirled around an accretion disk. Jets are present in the interstellar plasma. As dated back at 1918, astronomer H D Curtis saw a jet from the center of the M87 galaxy, describing it as a "curious straight ray" emanating from the galaxy. Taking the shape of a massive flashlight beam in space, a stream of electrons and protons moving at the speed of light can be seen in the NASA image of the galaxy. The jet is a strongly rotationally symmetric plasma beam (i.e. a coherent laser beam). Energetic astrophysical jets, with speeds approaching the speed of light, are seen on a variety of scales emerging from active galactic nucleus and young stars. They are thought to result from the dynamics of the accretion disks rotating around a large mass. Power radiates from charged particles traveling in a circular orbit (usually around a magnetic field associated with a jet).

Focused Light Beams from Rotating Chakras

The chakra is a revolving accretion disk on a fairly large, compact, subtle body. We also know (from the above discussion) that the nodes of the chakras are sites of strong magnetic fields, and the charged particles travel in helical or spiral paths around this field. Plasma magnetic fields are shifting with it. The effect of the movement of molecules, which plunges into the subtle body at high speed, is to effectively swirl the powerful magnet around the axis of the chakra cone. This causes the magnetic field to be twisted, raised and ejected as a jet of collimated light. The acceleration mechanism for most jets is magnetohydrodynamic. (Magneto- hydrodynamics provides a general structure for the study of the behaviors of magnetic plasma.) The jet being released should be parallel to the axis of rotation of the chakra.

Jets or guided light beams have been seen in photos taken during activities in which subtle energy practices (e.g. Reiki, Qigong and Christian 'Praise and Worship') take place. There are also Hindu, Buddhist Taoist, and Christian depictions depicting jets of light coming from the palms of saints and gods. The palms of the hands have broad chakras (and acupoints). The frequency and rotation rate of the chakra will have a direct effect on the strength and stability of the beam. One of the visionaries of the Fatima apparitions of "Mary," "Lucia," announced that during one of the apparitions, "Mary" had opened her hands and "rays of light" had poured out of them.

It can be achieved simply by changing the usual direction of the chakra spin (so that the energy is released rather than absorbed) and the rotational speed of the chakra in the palm (by consciously concentrating on the same chakra or acupoint in the palm of the hand). Jets can also be given from other chakras or acupoints such as from the heart chakra. For example, when Jesus appeared to St. Faustina, two light beams came out of his heart—one of the beams was blue and the other was red. Amusingly, jet formations in cosmic objects, such as galaxies, also show two light beams — one blue and the other red!

Black Holes and Chakras

Black holes, according to scientists, also cause jets. In fact, the M87 galaxy (cited above) which emits jets is suspected of harboring a black hole in its nucleus. (The black hole is then similar to the node and the galaxy to the cone form of the chakra.) This is frightening because, as far as we know, the intense gravitational fields of the black holes consume energy leaving little to escape. (Small black holes, however, send out Hawking radiation.) If we use the same theory as we did for the chakras, it might be because of the direction of spinning the accretion disks around the black holes. Does this refer to that if the direction of spinning the accretion disk of a rotating black hole ('Kerr') is reversed, it will start ejecting energy instead of consuming it? According to scientists, black holes with extremely energetic jets are the fastest to spin.

If we were to expand to black holes what we knew about the framework of the chakras, we would expect black holes to come in pairs. Every black hole will then be bound by a tube (popularly referred to as a "wormhole") that leads to another black hole in another part of our universe. This wormhole can be long or very small so that there is a double vortex structure (like in chakras) connected by a small tube-giving rise to jets ejecting astrophysical objects in opposite directions. Astrophysical jets moving in opposite directions of astrophysical bodies have been seen. We should also expect black holes to exist in all galaxies because they are simply points of entry into the network or web of "meridians" (in this case filamentary currents) that transfer energy from one point to another in the universe.

We are all energy beings and part of this magnificent universe. The colors of the chakras or the seven celestial energy centers in the body are linked to the colors of the rainbow: purple, indigo, blue, green, yellow, orange and red. As all colors combine into the purest white of the thousand-petalled lotus, so are the energy centers tuned to our supreme consciousness. Chakras are the key divine focal points of energy in the area of human vitality. Located along the core path of the body from the base of the spine to the highest point of the head, the chakras are accumulations of vital prana which are always in motion, balancing the resources and energy with the auras of the natural world.

Violet is the hue of the Crown Chakra, also known as Sahasrara, the seat of eternal consciousness and the light of the sky, where the conscious breath is falling into the boundless world of Shiva. This chakra is located at the highest point in the brain. The Crown Chakra is linked to the crown of the head, the sensory system, and the cerebral, illustrating pure thought and action, eternal, divine existence. This chakra associates one with the never-ending knowledge and the supernatural source. Opening this chakra will help to take advantage of a deep cosmic understanding where Shiva and Shakti merge as non-duality. Gemstone Mala Beads that help the Crown Chakra are sphatic or clear quartz beads.

Indigo: the shade of the Brow or the Third Eye Chakra, otherwise called Ajna. This chakra is situated between the temples of the hand, the location of the soul's unfolding. Wisdom and simple thinking or awareness free us from pain. To be able to clearly see your actions and those of others without prejudice, but with apathy, leads to the awakening of the Kundalini. We are who we are, and we are part of an inclusive manifesto. Opening this chakra will help clear up your intuition, your instinct and your trustworthiness. The Sapphire japa mala is connected to the Ajna Chakra.

Blue: Shadow of the Chakra throat, otherwise known as Visuddhi, is related to cleansing and balance that can be energized by pranayama or regulated breathing. This chakra is found in the throat or larynx where the vibrations of the sound are transformed into mantras. Just as mantras are healing vibrations and soothing, sorrowful words do harm not only to others but also to yourself. Control or balancing the throat chakra can contribute to spiritual purification, building outlets for great worldly communication. The opening of the Throat Chakra will enhance psychic hearing. Gemstone malas that will allow the Throat Chakra to integrate are turquoise, blue lapis and sodalite.

Green: the color of the Heart Chakra, better known as Anahata, where the subconscious unfolds and there is a gamut of emotions. This chakra is connected to the heart, the lungs, the circulatory system, and the cardiovascular plexus. The Heart Chakra conquers every barrier between the real and the infinite world. Realization and self-knowledge contribute to inner healing. Opening the Heart Chakra allows a man to love more, to sympathize, and to feel empathic. Gemstones yoga malas that will enable the heart chakra to integrate are emerald, tourmaline, aventurine, malachite and rose quartz.

Yellow: the color of the solar plexus chakra, otherwise known as Manipura. This chakra is located in the stomach zone and is a place of insight, wisdom, self-confidence and well-being. The seat of food couple with the digestion Manipuri Chakra is the fire of our soul, the sacred power. The vibrations from food are brought into our chakras, and here we have the power to remove negative thoughts. The Solar Plexus Chakra is an example of critical action and self-awareness. At a time when this chakra is open, it enables a man to locate his own quality, transforming dreams and objectives into reality. Gemstone mala beads and bracelets will support the Solar Plexus chakra to develop are gold, topaz, citrine, and yellow jasper.

Orange: the color of the Holy Chakra, otherwise known as Svadhisthan, is the seat of subconsciousness, between sleeping and waking, and is the triggering seat of the Karmas. This chakra is found between the coccyx and the sacrum. The Holy Chakra is linked to the sexual organs of procreation. Let go of the past, the ego that holds on to knowledge and judgmental behavior. This is where the Kundalini begins to develop. Opening this chakra will free the power of the will and the power of concentrated action. Gemstone yoga malas that will support the Sacral Chakra include fruit, jasper, coral, orange jade, and orange.

Red: the color of the Root of Chakra, otherwise known as the Muladhara, is the beginning of our spiritual evolution. This chakra is sited at the base of the spine and allows us to be ground where the kundalini shakti rests in a deep, passive state. The seat of the incapacitated, the root chakra, is where we begin to evaluate our reality and purify spiritual energy. Gemstone mala beads with yoga beads that will enable the Root Chakra to combine ruby, pomegranate, smoked quartz, obsidian, hematite and onyx.

There are major energy centers in every human body that are connected to the various organs and glands. Such energy centers are called chakras. Chakras are vibrating at a certain frequency, depending on which of the seven major chakras we're talking about. Chakras can be interpreted as a light spinning wheel, this spinning wheel behaves like a vortex and draws in any light that comes into contact with it, assuming that it is the same frequency of vibration. Chakras are often linked to different colors.

There are hundreds of small chakras or energy points all over the human body. These minor and seven major chakras draw information about the different frequency vibrations of our surroundings. Such knowledge may be the aura of another human, astral energy, or even something that gives off a vibrational frequency, which is all in modern physics. Bottom line, our chakras let us see how healthy our surrounding is. It includes the people and animals we come into contact with. Our chakras will also emit their own vibrational energy.

Each one of our seven major chakras is spiritually, emotionally, physically and mentally connected to us. The physical relation of the chakra regulates another glade or organ which, in turn, regulates another body part or feature of the body.

There is no organ, gland, or device in the body that is not related to the chakra. Then each chakra is related to a vibrational color frequency. To give you an example, the heart rate of the vibrational chakra is green. This chakra regulates the heart muscle, the lungs, the bronchial system, the lymph glands, the immune system, the secondary circulatory system along with the hands and arms.

These seven main chakras are aligned along the spinal column. The vitality level of the chakras will show any disturbances that may occur in the body, mind or spirit. In addition, each of the seven major chakras acts as its own intelligence processing center. This has a wide range of implications because it means that the chakra is not only linked to specific organs or glands but will also control aspects of our mental and emotional health.

The good news is that we can balance or tune our chakras. This is accomplished by introducing the vibrational color of the chakra, which is at the same frequency as the chakra that we want to balance. This can be done to help us improve our physical, mental, emotional and spiritual condition.

The human aura will resonate with the different colors of the chakras. If we understand what these colors mean, we have the knowledge we need to properly align our chakras.

CHAPTER TWO

Seven Major Types Of Chakras

Root

Root Chakra is known as the first of the seven. The Root Chakra is located at the bottom of the spine. This chakra is depicted in the color red, the first color of the rainbow. When the Root Chakra is functioning properly, the basic survival needs will be affected. These include caring for your family, housing, food, and making money. If this chakra isn't balanced, you can develop greed, not take care of and appreciate the things you have, develop a feeling of lack or need, and prevent you from maintaining your possessions and the surrounding.

One can balance the Root Chakra by placing a ruby or granite gemstone on that area and painting it charging the chakra with the positive reddish energy that swirls into that chakra in a clockwise motion. You can also clean the Root Chakra by making use of a black obsidian. Move the black obsidian over the Root Chakra in a counterclockwise direction, while picturing all the negative energy of the chakra swirling out into the stone.

Sacral

The second of the seven is the Holy Chakra. The Sacral Chakra is located at about the same level where the belly button is located. This chakra is represented in the color orange. The Sacred Chakra lends itself to a person's emotional state and creativity. When it's in balance, a person's creative side tends to come out that involves drawing, poetry, or any kind of art. If the Sacral Chakra isn't balanced, you can have mood swings.

The Sacral Chakra can be balanced in the same way that the Root Chakra is balanced. You may want to use a carnelian or a tiger's eye gemstone while attempting to balance it.

Solar Plexus

The third Chakra is the Solar Plexus is the of the seven chakras. The Solar Plexus Chakra is located just below the bottom of the ribs. This chakra is depicted in a yellow color. The Solar Plexus Chakra influences your activities and your energy. It also has a great impact on what you do and why you do it. When a person is healthy, he or she will develop a sense of wisdom about the activities they do. They tend to spend their time doing things that are worth doing. When the Solar Plexus

Chakra becomes unhealthful, people tend to become obsessed with certain areas of their lives. They could come, for example, a workaholic. They also tend to make poor decisions about what is the best course of action for their lives.

You should use calcite, amber or topaz honey when balancing the Solar Plexus Chakra. The balancing of the Solar Plexus Chakra is done in the same manner as the Root Chakra.

Heart

The fourth of the seven is the Heart Chakra. This Heart Chakra is located in the center of the chest and is depicted as green. In humans who have developed a deep love for their fellow man, the Heart Chakra will glow pink. The Heart Chakra reflects passion, relationships, and above all, affection. If you are safe, you will develop a sense of compassion for your fellow man, and you will be able to give and receive love and friendship with ease. The Heart Chakra also helps you to develop a sense of compassion for yourself. If the Heart Chakra is unhealthful, it can be difficult to find and maintain love and friendship. This can also be as a result of the fact that you close yourself off from others when the Heart Chakra is not safe.

You can balance your Heart Chakra with the use of jade and aventurine gemstones. Balancing the Heart Chakra can be done in the same way that the Root Chakra is balanced.

Throat

The Throat Chakra is widely considered as the fifth chakra of the seven chakras. The Throat Chakra is located at the bottom of the throat and is responsible for honest communication. The Throat Chakra is associated with the blue. When your Throat Chakra is healthy, your communication skills are good, and people can hear and understand what you have to say. It's also a very good chakra to be healthy if you're speaking in public. If it is not healthy, two areas of communication could develop. The first is that you tend to be overbearing in your manner of speech and talk too much. The next one is that you tend to be shy and don't talk a lot, thinking that what you say doesn't carry a lot of weight.

You can use blue lace agate or turquoise stones to balance the Throat Chakra. The Throat Chakra may be regulated in the same manner as the Root Chakra.

Brow

The Brow Chakra is the six of the seven. This chakra is linked to the third eye and the color is indigo. It is situated under the eyebrows and slightly upwards. The Brow Chakra is considered a chakra in which intelligence, psychic abilities and spirituality reside. When it is safe, your faith will come naturally to you, and you will appear to be confident with yourself. When the Brow Chakra is not safe, people appear to be closed-minded and have a problem concentrating.

You can use amethyst or lapis lazuli to balance the Brow Chakra. It can be aligned in the same way as the other Chakras.

Crown

The seventh chakra is the Crown Chakra. The Crown Chakra is like a crown on the top of the head. This chakra is represented by a purple color and sometimes a white color. You feel connected to the world and the universe when it's healthy. You also manage day-to-day disruptions well and are able to make short-term and long-term plans. When the Crown Chakra is unhealthful, you tend to make poor decisions when you are able to make decisions, and you may feel separate from the rest of the world.

You can balance the Crown Chakra with quartz and amethyst. You can also use quartz as a side note to complement any of the other chakras. It may be balanced in the same manner as the other chakras.

Healing with the Seven Major Chakras

Keeping the seven major chakras safe is necessary because we are actually moving slowly into another dimension of existence and, in order to do so, our bodies must achieve higher vibration and frequency ~ and this involves the awakening of five other major chakras that we have dormant right now; apart from the seven major chakras that we now know.

In order to ensure these five are awakened, the seven that we are now using must be in a healthy state of being.

ROOT CHAKRA

- The first center, between the thighs, around the sex organs.
- Gland: the suprarenal glands (cortisone, adrenaline, noradrenaline)
- The main color is red, and the secondary color is black.
- Main focus: SURVIVAL, GROUNDEDNESS, PHYSIQUE NEEDS.

To Be, To Have" is the keyword here. The smells are sandalwood and vetiver. An open and balanced Root Chakra allows for the required grounding (earth and nature support) of strong structural elements of the physical body; adrenals, spinal column, kidneys, lungs, bones, teeth, thighs, knees, lower back, hair, large intestine, pelvic region and smooth operation of the excretory system. The Root Chakra binds us to the ground, takes control of the hands and knees, the sciatic nerve and the consistency of the blood. Allergic reactions are also related to the Root Chakra.

When one has a strong Root Chakra, one stands firmly on the ground with both feet. It concerns one's will to live, one's sense of security, one's instincts and basic communication, concerns related to food, clothing, shelter-practical things, self- preservation, endurance, rhythm and connection to nature, etc.

SACRAL CHAKRA

- Second center; lower abdomen to navel.

- Gland: the gonades. Testicles and ovaries (testosterone and estrogen)
- The color is brown.
- Main focus: VITALITY, CREATIVITY, DESIRE, SELF-WORTH.
- "To Feel, To Desire," is crucial.
- The scents are ylang ylang and patchouli.

A well-developed Sacral Chakra ensures the health of the reproductive system: testicles, penis, ovaries and uterus, duodenum, ileum, cecum, lower vertebrae, small intestine, pelvis, urinary tract and bladder. It also prevents impotence and decreases menstrual pain. A strong Sacral Chakra helps to assimilate food, to detoxify the body and to strengthen the immune system. Potency, procreation, fertility and healthy sexual activity, vitality, creativity, joy of living, harmonious relationships and work with others, surrender, tolerance, movement, giving and receiving, all depend on a healthy chakra.

SOLAR PLEXUS CHAKRA

- Third center; about 4 "above the navel
- Gland: pancreas (insulin, digestive enzymes)
- Its color is yellow.
- Key focus: WILLFULNESS, JOY, ENERGY.
- "To Do, To Act," is key.
- Scents are grapefruit and fennel.
- Also known as the Navel Chakra.

Those with an open and balanced Solar Plexus Chakra may have awesome appetites and make optimum use of nourishment taken in, have good body temperature regulation, are radiant, seldom complain of problems with liver, stomach, or any other digestive organs, sleep deeply, have steady nerves, handle stress well and can master their desires, with a great sense of humor and laughter. Problems with the third chakra result in eating disorders such as anorexia or obesity - center around psychic problems related to the Navel Chakra, and many other issues rooted in the stomach or digestive system, such as diseases of the liver, heartburn, spleen or gall bladder, nervous disorders, obesity, backache, anorexia, etc.

HEART CHAKRA

- 4th center; the center of the chest at heart level.
- Gland: Thymus (immune system)
- Main color is green and secondary is pink.
- Key focus: LOVE, TRUST, COMPASSION.
- "To Love, To Be Loved."
- Scents: Rose Geranium and Rose Otto.

Beings with a strong Heart Chakra have a lot of love, may have compassion for all of humanity, forgiveness, peace, understanding, compassion, group consciousness, acceptance and contentment.

THROAT CHAKRA

- 5th center; larynx, throat area.
- Gland: thyroid and parathyroid (thyroxine)
- Its representative color is sky blue.
- Key focus: COMMUNICATIONS, LISTENING, VIBRATIONS.
- "To Speak, Hear and Be Heard."
- Scents are Bergamote, Spruce.

This is the hearing and speaking center. A rich sound of one's voice is the sound of a healthy Throat Chakra. One breathes freely and will not ordinarily experience any inflammation or tonsillitis.

THIRD EYE CHAKRA

- 6th center; middle of the forehead.
- Gland: Pituitary (vasopressin)

- The symbolic color is indigo/dark blue.
- Main focus: PSYCHIC ABILITIES, INTUITION, CONNECTING with HIGHER SELF.
- "To See, Self-Knowledge."
- Scents: lavender and basil
- Also known as the Forehead Chakra.

Those with well-developed Third Eye chakras may have expanded cognitive skills, clairvoyance, enhanced analytical ability, peace of mind, perception beyond duality, wisdom, great imagination and visualization skills, healing energy, mental clarity, self-confidence, remarkable powers of concentration, great intelligence, and vision and hearing are sharp even in old age.

The Forehead Chakra directly relates to the pituitary gland which is the main control center of the entire endocrine system, regulating the activity of all endocrine glands, the hormonal system, cerebellum, eye, nose, ears, sinuses, inner ears/eyes, mental neurological abilities, hearing/sight, and hypothalamus, influencing the immune system and nervous systems and in the end, one's psychological constitution. Emotional connections to this chakra also involve self- awareness, cognitive intelligence, sureness, mental balance, etc.

CROWN CHAKRA

- The seventh center; the top of the head.
- Gland: Pineal (serotonin, melatonin) T
- The symbolic color is purple. The second color is white.
- Key focus: Peace, Knowledge, THE GATEWAY.
- "I Learn, Cosmic Consciousness."
- Scents: neroli and frankincense.

A healthy Crown Chakra promotes good health by supporting the body's own natural healing mechanisms, but if it is blocked, it may lead to serious illness. The Crown Chakra is the brain, the pineal gland, and the entire nervous system. The pineal gland reacts to light and regulates sleep rhythms. This center of awareness is for the universal consciousness, the union of the higher self with the soul, harmony with the Source, spiritual will, inspiration, Divine wisdom and understanding, idealism, selfless service, knowledge beyond space and time, spirituality, enlightenment and self- realization.

Blockages/weakness in the Crown Chakra can lead to headaches, weak immune system, nervous system, paralysis, multiple sclerosis, mental confusion, forgetfulness, cancer, mental illness, depression, chronic illness, lack of inspiration, sleep disorders, confusion, alienation, hesitancy, depression, senility, etc.

As you can see, the chakras have essential functions and they should be kept in a harmonious balance. Healing your chakras can be done by yourself, by someone else in person or remotely when they are trained and/or experienced in this skill. No matter how you choose, it's important because of the ever-increasing urgency of maintaining the health of our chakras.

You don't even have to be the type that can feel the energy moving in order to reap the benefits of the adjustments that will be made. Don't let your disbelief stop you from taking this important step in improving the healing of your mental, physical, and spiritual self.

The third chakra is located on the solar plexus. This is the core of personal power, will, self-expression, and other decisions. Fire is the element associated with the third chakra. Fire is a symbol of forward motion, manifestation, self-expression. Fire is also associated with the body's hot processes, digestion and metabolism.

Power is the force that blocks or interferes with the third chakra. This may be the client's own judgments that say that their lives should look a certain way and fit into nice, neat boxes. Finally, in the sixth, I saw pictures of the filing cabinets. A rigid idea (judgment) of what and how you should be limits self-expression and also contains an element of fear. I often see the energy of others seeking to influence or exploit the client. This energy can have the quality of despair if it comes from someone who's afraid, they might be left behind and they're trying to hold on to it. It can also have an edge or an unpleasant quality if it's from someone who really tries to exploit it. I also see this in the form of cords from one individual to another. The interesting thing is that these cords can come from physical and non-physical beings, from present and past lives.

To explain this, think of situations where a lot might have been achieved by usurping the personal power or will of a person. Perhaps the person had, or has, a talent that could make money for someone in authority over them. Another example could be arranged marriages, not only did the parents have complete control of the daughter, but also the husband they wanted for her. The energy from these previous experiences can stay with a person and limit their self-expression in this lifetime. Feelings of frustration or futility about finding your place in the world, intense self-judgment, or lack of self-confidence can indicate the blocks in this chakra. The good news is that blocks can be identified and cleared up.

The outgoing or Yang feature of the third chakra is the representation of the world's self. The receptive or Yin function of the third chakra concerns opinions and judgments about oneself and others.

In my view, the third chakra is the center from which you manifest your life as a divine being in a physical body on this earth plane. It is also the nucleus through which you manifest your wishes and your intentions. Will and confidence look a lot the same to me. The energy associated with the third chakra is the mind, ideas and thoughts that are the beginning of the manifestation.

When the third chakra is working properly, we experience the quality of expansiveness within ourselves. We feel that we belong, and we feel that we have something to offer the world. Yellow represents the color of the third chakra.

There is a great deal of people who seek healing methods, some of which are based on Eastern (not entirely geographical) practices such as yoga, chi quong or tai chi. There are spiritual practices and customs around the world, in different cultures and systems of faith with the same text. We have the ability and power to heal ourselves, to experience the interconnectedness with the world, if only we can sit still and listen to our inner voices, our inner guidance.

There is a culture of the heart. There is an age of imagination and compassion to come. The heart plays a starring role in this new age. Healthy meditation of the heart

Healing the chakras to release the toxic effects of daily stress is believed to be popularized by the New Age Movement. These energy centers can help bring balance to life, make us feel more positive and help to release the toxins that we accumulate in our daily lives. The meditation, opening and balancing of the chakras help to activate this energy center.

The Root Chakra is located at the bottom of the spine; two inches below the belly button is the Sacral Chakra. Between the belly button and base of the ribcage is the Solar Plexus, in the middle, between the breasts is the Heart Chakra, next is the Throat Chakra, between the eyebrows is the famous Third Eye and at the top of the head is the Crown Chakra.

The Heart Chakra

The heart is where we live our passions. It's fragile and easily broken, but it's wonderfully resilient. There's no point trying to fool the heart. It depends on our honesty to survive.

The heart is the center of love, the energy system of man. Is love healing everyone? Who didn't feel the pain of a broken heart, grief and sorrow, the devastating effect of betrayal, emotional problems, abandonment, rejection and separation – just to name a few in a long list of hurtful situations? It takes more than physical healing to dry up the tears of the wounded heart. If neglected, the pain of the heart affects the spirit, the energy drains, the mind, the body and the spirit are disconnected. More often than not, medical treatment is not enough to cure heart problems.

Believe it or not, we're all connected to the Divine. We have the gift of perception, the gift of thinking, of understanding. We just need to know how to tap into these talents to see us through the hard times and to enjoy the good times. Is faith blind enough? Not all of us are ready to believe, much less open our minds to find that deeper connection to the Divine.

The Heart Chakra is situated in the center of your chest, in Sanskrit it is the Anahata Chakra, which means unstuck. It is linked and connected to the physical and spiritual self. It's the mid-point of our physical bodies. This lies between the three lower chakras that keep us going in the physical realm. The Heart Chakra at the upper layer is the three upper chakras that help us to grow in the spiritual realm where our intuition, thoughts, imagination, and creativity can be realized.

Chakra believers, calming and balancing the energies of the key chakras, claim that this leads to healing of dis-ease, opens up the intuitive abilities with which we are born, calms the mind and paves the way for inner peace. We learn how to let life run, to be more appreciative of the countless riches of which we are blind. We come to realize that problems and anxieties do not need to dominate our waking hours, thus tormenting the subconscious.

We understand and embrace the value of love through the Heart Chakra – the unconditional love that is available to us all. As the Heart Chakra spreads, it includes the other six major chakras, bringing the physical and the spiritual self into harmony, bringing life into balance. Meditating with the Heart

Chakra expands the meaning of thoughts, words and deeds — it moves us into the true meaning of love — a universal and unconditional love.

The Heart Chakra radiates strength that allows us to live a full and fulfilling life. It's a guiding force that connects the physical and spiritual planes that help us avoid being self-centered, uncaring, feeling like a victim, and other features. The Heart Chakra is the center where we attract abundance in our lives, so we can share it with others. We share a world beyond ourselves, we move beyond the clear boundaries of our physical world, we become more aware that we are all connected. It's easier to say than to do it.

There are a lot of meditation forms. Working with the chakras is a process of meditation and visualization. There are sites on the internet that deliver strong meditation practice in the Heart Chakra. Meditation is your personal choice.

Every being that inhabits this universe is made up of energy! This energy is electromagnetic, and each being has a slightly different wavelength. Have you ever heard someone say, "You 're on my wavelength?" We have a physical body, a mind and a soul. There is also another very significant dimension to the being, the Hara. This is the center of emotions, and it has a unique energy within us. There are layers and strata of energy to the body, and the Hara is nearest to the center of the Central

Star. We are all energetically focused on the Heart Chakra, the core of our emotional selves. "The Chakras are spinning vortexes of energy in the being and are full of colored light. We are light beings! Each chakra is aligned with the aspect of the being and can be energized to heal the body, mind and soul. They act as sheaths of energy over the whole being, including the center, the Hara and the Aura!

To add joy to your life, the Hara and Heart Chakra must be healed of all negative emotions. To bring healing to any of these, you can use the Rose Quartz crystal, which has strong effects on the pain we have endured and allows us to love ourselves again. Through holding the crystal in the left hand and experiencing the energy flowing through the being, we will heal. You can also heal by energizing the Heart Chakra by meditation.

By feeling the energy of your heart flowing through you and focusing on energy, you can energize the Heart Chakra! Using positive affirmations such as "I Love My World!" It would help a lot! Since this chakra is green in color and the best way to bring this color to your life is by walking in nature where you can see the green grass and the green leaves on the trees.

The Heart Chakra will also energize the other Chakras, pray in meditation that your heart would protect your life, and the Solar Plexus Chakra will be enabled! The statement here would be, "I protect my soul!" As the presence of the being that protects us, the brighter this chakra, the more protected you will feel. The chakra color is yellow, and by introducing yellow into your life by clothing, home decoration or consuming yellow food, you will help to energize! Spring can be a good time for this color in nature, as there are many yellow flowers around.

By praying the heart will nurture your being, the Sacred Chakra will be activated! Please pray the affirmation of your own world here, such as, "I nurture my relationship with my family and friends!" I will nurture my children! "I love my pets and garden that belongs to me." The center of our nurturing aspect is the color orange, which is also related to creativity, and so perhaps another assertion to add would be "I feel creative." Try to plant orange flowers in your garden or as houseplants and bring orange into your life!

To activate the Root Chakra, the grounding energy of Mother Earth, you need to pray that your heart is loving Mother Earth, affirming that "I love the Great Mother Earth!" The color of this chakra is red and it is a strong color. Too much is not recommended at home in Feng Shui, so keep it to soft shades of red such as scarlet or burgundy. It is a good idea to add features such as roses in a vase or other flowers or to visit poppies in the field.

You always begin to activate the chakras by grounding yourself, by working through the lower chakras. Now we can begin to activate the higher chakras to reach the Universe, the next is the Throat Chakra, this is the vital aspect of communication, and by praying to communicate with love and understanding, you will find this chakra energized. "The best way to bring the color of this turquoise chakra into your life is by looking at the sky!"

The Brow Chakra is the center of mindful awareness of the being, and the mind has two aspects, logic and thought and intuition – different kinds of consciousness, all of which are important to the being. To activate this chakra, you need to pray that you think and feel in love and make the same statement, "I think and feel in love!" The indigo color is a lovely color to have around your home, and as this is the color of the Brow Chakra, it will help to energize it.

The Crown Chakra is relative to your prayers and your spirituality. It is quite easy to activate this chakra by praying that my spirituality is love. It will be a good reinforcement of the same. It would be violet to introduce the color of the chakra into your life. Flowers, clothes, or decorations, or even a purple veil on the window to shine purple light into the room, would be a good thing.

The fifth chakra is in the throat. This is the center of communication and it is linked to the soul for the purpose of expressing its desires. In my experience, the work of the fifth chakra is much deeper than simple communication. We speak our truth via the fifth chakra and convey who we are, what we are here for and what we want. Cyndi Dale says the fifth function is "the ability to know ourselves in the world." This is not even easy to do, because the energy behind this expression is conviction and conviction comes from a sense of dignity and value. Invalidation and indignity are the energies that block the fifth chakra.

It may have been impossible in this lifetime or in previous lifetimes to speak your truth out of fear of punishment, persecution, or even death. This energy may be absolutely irrational in this present life, but the fear it gives rise to is real and shuts it down to the communication center.

A whole other energy that blocks the fifth chakra is to judge or censor or swallow your words to accept them, whether it's good or not for you in the end. I'm not talking about being socially acceptable I'm talking about not being true to myself in order to be "good" to another person or group of people.

The fifth chakra is a vehicle to process and release emotions. "Talking it out" is a great description of the healing effect of talking through your feelings, which releases them from your physical body.

The outgoing or Yang purpose of the fifth chakra is to convey it verbally. The receptive or Yin feature of the fifth chakra is linked to obtaining guidance.

The fifth Chakra is the gap between the basic four lower chakras (6th) and the mind (7th). This chakra is the ether or space where four elements are present. Peter Rendel explained in his book *"Introduction to the Chakras"* that the fifth Chakra: "On this (throat) level, we feel the quality of space alone."

We have seen that the four lower elements all have qualities that are activities in space. Ether is the space itself within which these activities take place. The sound sense comes from the ether dimension.

Everything is energy, every person, every emotion, every thought, and all that energy makes an imprint. It's all in the walls, in the fixtures, in the furniture. By cleaning up this energy, everything is brought into the present day, and a clean slate is rendered so that room is opened up to those who live there and allow those who work there. It's necessary to clean up the ancient energy of the enterprises.

The walls, the doors and the appliances are all there. By clearing this energy, it all enters the present time and a clean slate is made so that space can take up and empower those who live and work there. In the case of companies, to make room for new clients, it is important to clear out the old energy of customers. It is important for everyone's well-being, as everyone is affected by others' energies.

The seven major chakras are linked to positions along your spine. The first of the chakras, the Root Chakra, is located at the bottom of the tailbone, the second chakra or the Sacral Chakra is about two inches below the naval. The third chakra or the Solar is on the solar plexus. The fourth chakra or Heart is in the middle of the chest, the fifth chakra or Throat is at the base part of the neck, the sixth Chakra or Brow (sometimes called the Third Eye) is at the center of the head, behind the eyes, and the seventh chakra is at the top of the head. All but the seventh chakra can be visualized as a rotating vortex passing through the body, back and forth.

The chakras cover a wide spectrum from fully physical to spiritual at the first chakra: the seventh chakra is the key to the heart. They have an influence on every aspect of life.

This section is dedicated to the first chakra or the Root Chakra. Located on the tip of the tail bone, it is closest to the earth. The element attributed to the root chakra is the earth. This is the chakra from which we have grounded. The mission is to send and receive energy from the earth. So, by consciously grounding it, we are stabilizing our physical body, aligning our chakras and creating a vehicle to release unprofitable energy.

When we are overwhelmed or scattered, our consciousness is not in our bodies. "Ground" is the solution. Grounding takes you into the present moment because it puts you into the body. If you feel out of control or overwhelmed or scattered, take a minute to create a grounding cord, and you'll immediately shift your energy. You can ground by mere imagining a colored beam of light stretching from the tip of your tailbone to the middle of the earth. Actually, there's more to it than that, and I know there are a lot of people who have difficulty grounding.

The first chakra is characterized by physicality; being in the body, health, survival, loving relationships, passion, struggle or flight. It's also about feeling safe and secure, so issues about money, not feeling protected or looking to someone else for your safety and validation can affect the first chakra.

The first chakra receives its basic programming from the family, and there may be limited information and "programs" from the parents remaining in the first chakra. Our parents were responsible for our survival as children, and they gave us information like "don't talk to strangers" to keep us safe. Although this is good advice for children, if it's still a belief that you hold as an adult, you may be missing out on a great conversation with very cool people. Your parents have given you what they knew. So, if they struggled with money or health, they 're most likely to pass it on to you as well. Believing in "It's hard to get ahead" or "save your money for a rainy day" has nothing to do with your present life, but it may be part of your energetic body that either keeps prosperity away or makes it very difficult to enjoy for fear that it might be taken away at any moment.

Most of the time, this energy is fear that has built a foothold in lifetimes where basic physical survival is at risk, lifetimes where hunger, sickness, or physical danger is prevalent. This is totally irrational in this lifetime, but it can affect a healthy relationship with food or cause anxiety or worry that people are out to hurt you or have you convinced that you are supposed to have a disease. This kind of energy can have an impact on you throughout your life. It's like being held prisoner by something you can't explain, but it's a very real feeling.

The first chakra is also where mothers are linked to their young children. Children rely on their mother to survive and to show them how to survive. These strings exist until around the age of seven or eight when the child becomes more independent.

When the first chakra is working properly, you feel strong and vital. You know that you have the right to be loved and the right to be successful in your life. You have your foundation, so to speak. You can sit in a quiet place and know that you know that you're safe and that you can handle anything that's going on in your life. The color associated with the first chakra is red, the most concentrated color in the spectrum.

Chakras Location

The chakras have a particular location linked to the physical body and listed below is this information, plus the Sanskrit name of each chakra. Only the most important chakras are featured. The body has several major and minor chakras, but I'm going to concentrate on the key chakras in this section. Every chakra also has a specific number of spokes or petals, which signify the primary and secondary force of undulation as the energy enters the depression in the etheric body where the chakra is located.

Center No.1 Basic or Root; Location: at the base of the spine; Sanskrit Name: Muladhara; No. of Spokes/Petals: 4

Center No.2 Sacral; location: sex organs; Sanskrit Name: Svadhishthan; No. of Spokes/Petals: 6

Center No.2 Spleen; Location: over physical spleen; Sanskrit Name: Nil; No. of Spokes/Petals: 6

Center No.3 Navel or Solar Plexus Chakra; Location: located in the area of the navel and solar plexus; Sanskrit Name: Manipura; No. of Spokes/Petals: 10.

Center No.4 Heart; Location: over the physical heart; Sanskrit Name: Anahata; No. of Spokes/Petals: 12.

Center No.5 Throat; location: at the front of the throat; Sanskrit Name: Vishuddha; No. of Spokes/Petals: 16.

Center No.6 Third Eye; location: between the eyebrows; Sanskrit Name: Ajna; No. of Spokes/Petals: 96.

Center No.7 Crown; Location: at the top of the head; Sanskrit Name: Sahasrara; No. of Spokes/Petals: 972

The Lower Centers:

No. 1 and 2 have very few petals and are mainly based on obtaining the 'serpent-fire' from the earth (Centre 1) and the energy from the sky (Centre 2 - the spleen). The chart above has two chakras represented as second centers. Within the Hindu tradition, the second center is represented by the Sacred Chakra, but the teachings of theosophy do not promote the activation of the Sacred Chakra and tend to represent the spleen as the second center.

The Middle Centers:

No. 3, 4 and 5 are those who are related to human personality. The powers involved are lower Astral (Centre 3), higher Astral (Centre 4) and lower Mind/Manas (Centre 5).

All these feeds the central nervous system and are profoundly involved in the Physical Plane of Life and how man forms his personality and lives on the earth's surface.

The Higher Centers

No. 6 and 7 only come into action when a certain amount of spiritual awareness has been developed by the human being. No. 6 is linked and connected to the Pituitary Gland and No. 7 to the Pineal Gland.

The number of spokes or petals reflects the quality of the energy center and its primary focus. The goal is to pump the energy into the higher chakras, but the incoming energy would naturally affect the chakras that have the most impact within the human psyche. The primary incoming force is undulated over and under the particular consistency of each of the spokes, and each of them is determined by the features of the chakra. For example, the heart chakra is associated with commitment, charity, loyalty, and other similar attributes, and the heart chakra is subdivided into those characteristics.

Secondary incoming energy is further influenced by the creation of positive or negative qualities associated with the chakra. The incoming energy is strengthened or weakened, depending on the power of the force that passes through the spokes.

To explain briefly, the higher chakras are better than the lower or middle chakras. The number of spokes/petals in the chakra reflects the spiritual growth of the energy center; further speaking, the chakra grows spiritually. However, within each chakra, the spokes/petals have a further filter system.

The down-pouring of divine energy is limitless, but what we can absorb depends upon our chakras' creation. If the dominant ones are our lower chakras, then this is how much energy we get from primary and secondary powers of energy.

You have to make sure the higher chakras rule your life most if you want to become more spiritual. Since high chakras are mainly influenced by compassion, peace and the like, all you need to do is live your life in these parameters.

CHAPTER THREE

Our Lives As A Reflection Of Our Chakras

The emphasis made in this book is on the personalities of the different chakras and how easy it is to understand them and to balance them. It is necessary to open and stabilize the energy centers, since this allows the energy to flow freely up and down the column and the nervous system. It often results in a sense of peace and goodness because the physical, mental, emotional and spiritual bodies are directly associated with the system of the chakra. The chakras can emit tension, negative emotions and other imbalanced energies, which can support the person as a whole, as all the bodies are connected since all chakras are connected with the entire chakra network when one area works.

Qualities of the Chakras

First Chakra - Red: some of its qualities are inspiration, zeal, power and energy. Red helps to give us vitality, courage, inner strength and self-confidence and encourages us to achieve our goals. It gives us the strength and power to fulfill our dreams.

Second Chakra - Orange: it's linked to our emotions and self-feeling, and some of its qualities are joy, happiness and sociability.

Third Chakra - Yellow: this is our ego core and some of its strengths are confidence, intellect, and mental imagination. The heart is very much influenced by this chakra.

Fourth Chakra - Green: the Solar Plexus Chakra is the energy clearing center of the house. It is assumed that a significant portion of the energy from the lower chakras passes through this front chakra before entering the higher chakras and vice versa. The entire body can be enhanced by energizing this chakra. This chakra is linked to our loving self. Some of its qualities are harmony, empathy, emotional balance, compassion, unconditional love, understanding and development.

Fifth Chakra - Blue: the Throat Chakra is linked to our expressive self. Some of its qualities include honesty, politeness, creative self-expression and will. It also helps us to plan and organize in detail.

Sixth Chakra - Indigo: this chakra is also referred to as the master chakra because the other chakras and endocrine glands are directed and controlled. It is also popularly called the Third Eye because it is aligned with our simple self-search. Weisheit, seeking the truth and intuition are some of the features.

Seventh Chakra - Violet: this chakra is linked to our spiritual selves and intellect. Many of the virtues are creativeness, charisma and a desire to experience and to see the beauty of life which also develops our creative and artistic skills.

Many techniques are available to clear, balance and energize the chakras, but I'm going to give you a few simple techniques that everyone can utilize.

First technique: shake your hands to expel old energy and rub your hands rapidly. This will activate the smaller chakras in your legs, and the energy will pass. They could feel warm. First, put both hands on the chakra that you want to work with. Imagine the universal healing energy coming into your hands as you set out to clear, balance and energize the chakra you have your hands on. You can feel the heat going into that region as it happens. Continue for a few minutes or until you feel like it's over. When you're done, shake off the steam. Repeat the next chakra procedure.

Second Technique: it might be better if you lay down. Shake your hands to clear up the energy, then rub it quickly together.

Next, open both hands, palms down, one on top of the other. Place both hands over the chakra that you are working with and start circling counterclockwise about 3 to 5 inches above the chakra. Make slow counterclockwise circles over the chakra for about 1 to 2 minutes or until you feel it's finished.

Next, shake your hands and wind in a clockwise direction for half the time. Moving in the clockwise direction calms the cleared chakra and stabilizes it. For each chakra, repeat the same process. Clear the crown chakra in the right direction for a person to clear it and then in the left direction to soften it. The other chakras are the same as the above.

You can periodically or whenever you feel the need to use these techniques. Start the area where you feel uncomfortable. As mentioned above, the increasing chakra has its own characteristics. Look at the particular areas that cause your inconvenience, including the Heart Chakra.

This process may result in toxic or blocked energies that will then be able to move out of your body. When we express ourselves through these energy centers, once cleared of anxiety and negative feelings, we will move into a healthier state of well-being. Remember that all the chakras are linked, so clearing one will have an effect on the others as well. The clearing of the chakras will boost your entire energy system.

How Chakras Affect Our Psychic Minds

When the chakras are clean and healthy, energy flows freely through the body. We experience disease in the body when our chakras are unbalanced. As all mind or body or spirit systems are connected and interrelated, disease in one field will facilitate disease in others.

When we keep our chakras balanced and clean, we support our physical, mental, emotional and spiritual health. Clear and balanced chakras foster a clear psychic mind. Cleansing with balancing the chakras can be done by prayer, intention, visualization and by calling upon non-physical beings such as Michael and Archangels Metatron as well as Melchizedek (master of the Judaic and New Age).

Increasing chakra is associated with major nerve ganglia branching out of the spinal column. In addition, the chakras are also correlated with the levels of consciousness, the archetypal elements, the evolutionary stages of life, colors, sounds and functions of the body. These are the chakras:

Root Chakra = Earth, Physical Being, Self- Preservation - Red

Located at about the base of the spine, this chakra is our foundation. It is connected to our survival instincts (food, shelter, money, etc.), our sense of being grounded, and our relation to our physical bodies. When this chakra is safe, it attracts wealth, prosperity and security.

Sacra Chakra = Emotional Identity, Self-Gratification Orange

Located a few inches above the Root Chakra (lower back, sexual organs) this chakra is linked to emotions and sexuality. This binds us to others through thoughts, wishes, sensations and movements. When we're safe, this chakra gives us fluidity, grace, sexual satisfaction, and the willingness to embrace change.

Solar Plexus Chakra = Fire, Identity of the Ego, Self- Identity - Yellow

Located in the solar plexus region, this chakra concerns personal strength, will, autonomy and metabolism. When we're safe, this chakra gives us strength, performance, spontaneity and uncontrollable power.

Heart Chakra = Air, Social Identity, Self-Acceptance - Green

This chakra is situated near to the heart and is linked to love in the center of seven chakras. The member is also the male and female, light and shadow, ego and unity integrator. This

Chakra helps us to love deeply, experience compassion and a deep sense of peace and concentration if we are well.

Throat Chakra = Sound, Creative Identity, Self- Expression – Blue

Located at the throat, this chakra is related to communication and innovation. Here, symbolically, we experience the world through sound, such as words.

Brow/Third Eye Chakra = Light, Archetypal Name, Self-Reflection - Indigo

Located between the eyes, this chakra is linked to the physical and intuitive process of seeing. It opens up our psychic faculties and understanding of archetypal levels. When we're healthy, this chakra helps us to see clearly- which allows us to see a "big picture."

Crown Chakra = Thinking, Universal Identity, Self- Knowledge – Violet

Located and situated at the top of the head, this chakra refers to consciousness as pure knowledge. It's our relation to the place of All-

Knowing. When created, this chakra brings knowledge, understanding, wisdom, spiritual connection and bliss to us.

Our mind/body/spirit links are openly connected from one to the other when our chakras are balanced. This movement makes our mental mind more responsive. In addition to feeling much better, we get a clearer and more reliable spiritual and intuitive awareness.

How to Balance Our Minds with the Root Chakra

Are you struggling with your entire frame of mind, which seems to be spacey and disorganized? Are you easily controlled by strong feelings of anger over simple things? Do you feel that your trust and drive have been thrown out of the window and that you can no longer focus on your goals? Chances are you really need root chakra balancing to restore lost trust in place of fear, calm in place of rage, and drive in place of pessimism. Chakras, particularly the Root Chakra, are stunning yet somewhat complicated. The Root Chakra is the ultimate foundation of another chakra, and if it is unbalanced, other chakras will follow suit.

Why do you align your root or foundation chakra? First and foremost, imagine the red color that glows at the end of your spinal cord, where this energy center is located. Starting with simple meditation, you need to see a bright red light at the base of your spinal cord. This is the ultimate start of cleansing and balancing your Root Chakra. Another good way to balance this chakra is by dancing. If you're not a good and passionate dancer, then this is the perfect opportunity to improve your dancing skills, and physical activity is a great way to release your endorphins and collect your feel-good energy. It's better to sing along to the music you're dancing to, as it helps to balance your throat chakra as well.

Yoga is an excellent remedy if you want to align every chakra, including your Root Chakra. There are quite a number of yoga postures that are ultimate for the cleansing and balancing of the root chakra. Some of these yoga poses, such as the tree posture, go hand in hand with the red visualization procedure. The tree pose is extremely helpful in balancing the Root Chakra, particularly if you focus on this meditation and form a single-handed tree pose. Ensure you feel sufficiently connected to the earth when performing this yoga pose, and don't forget to engage your core.

Surprisingly, taking a shower is an amazing Root Chakra cleaner. It is important to love and fully embrace your physical being by taking a shower. Mindfulness is a superb form of meditation, especially for your Root Chakra. After a satisfactory shower, a walk outside can improve the balance of your Root Chakra. Taking a thoughtful walk while concentrating deeply on every step you take will give this energy center a fantastic opportunity to clean up itself. In addition, paying attention to every step you take will give your mind a break from distracting thoughts or issues that may trigger stress and allow your Root Chakra to relax.

As with all seven major chakras, imbalances and blockages are diverse and, in some situations, individuals can benefit from chakra calming sessions with skilled energy healers. Trained Reiki Masters and even courses are available on virtual platforms to inform and provide free resources to those interested in maintaining their chakras. In many cases, the imbalance of the Root Chakra may spread or affect the function of other energy centers. Gifted psychic advisers may be able to help identify the underlying factors associated with the chakra system when individuals suffering from the imbalance would otherwise not have known the source of their dysfunction, which often leads to a worsening condition.

Having a massage can be the best way to balance your Root Chakra. Feeling good about your physical self will bring back the lost confidence and drive. Exploring and realizing the beauty of our physical self can help to clear out the incriminating feeling of anger and fear that causes uncertainty and other feelings of adversity caused by such variations in the imbalanced Root Chakra, thus balancing the energy center together. Balancing the root chakra is just like building a strong foundation for your house. Keep the Root Chakra balanced, and you're sure you'll have a healthy, balanced, open chakra system.

Where does energy originates?

According to the teachings of the chakras, the energy shaping what we call life energy originates in two chakras: sensual love in the sacral chakra and spiritual, eternal love in the heart chakra. The union of the two chakras increases the full potential of human love.

The Power of Love

The power of love transforms the world through emotional awareness, through the capacity for wisdom, compassion, practical support, and caring thoughts. Love is bringing about a multitude of positive changes. Love brings more happiness to the world. Those who do little, daily things with love take more pleasure in doing them. It reduces the misery of the earth. The power of love overcomes the power of hate and violence. This gives more awareness to the world. We really only know what we see through the eyes of the heart. The power of love is touching everything. You can increase your success in the material world by doing what you do with love. When your deeds are permeated with the power of love, you will be more successful in everything you do.

What could be done with the power of love

You can heal emotional wounds and release blockages with the power of love. When you call to mind old emotional wounds and cover them with a mental image of love, you will find that they disappear and that new powers are built up within you.

How can you make use of the power of love?

You can use the power of selfless love to create a closer bond with your fellow human beings and to achieve happiness in life. Visualize the people you have problems with and let the power of love flow through your image. You'll notice that you feel great and more relaxed and happier about them. You will brighten the sun by meditating on the power of love and radiating love to the universe. As a result, you won't lose energy, but instead, you will gain it. Because the power of love is so important, it is good for us to let this power rise and grow within us. When you focus on your chakras, you do it anyway. Through removing blockages in your sacral and heart chakras, you increase the power of love, by which you can once again achieve a state in which your Heart and Sacral Chakras harmonize with each other. Here are some activities to support this process.

Exercise

Harmonizing your heart and your sacred chakras. It's best to sit in a half-lotus position for this exercise, but the most important thing is that you feel comfortable. The more you use this technique, the more effective it is. You can do it when you're sitting on a chair on the subway, when you're lying in bed, and when you're walking. In order for this exercise to be a success, it is important that neither your Heart Chakra nor your Sacred Chakra is strongly blocked. If that's the case, focus on loosening chakra blockages.

Sit back, in the place of the lotus, if possible. Relax and breathe in and out a couple of times. Put your right hand (if male) or your left hand (if female) on your chest above your heart chakra and the other hand on your lower abdomen, below your navel, above the Sacral Chakra. Close your eyes gently. When you inhale, imagine the energy is flowing from your Sacral Chakra to your Heart Chakra, and when you exhale, the energy current is moving from your heart chakra to your Sacral Chakra.

Exercise for a total of seven inhalations and exhalations.

Now change the location of your hands, without touching your palms on your body. Shift your hands from one chakra to another in a semi-circle. The lower hand now crosses over your core chakra and the upper hand below your Sacral Chakra.

Inhale and imagine the energy flow from your Heart Chakra to your Sacral Chakra and, as you exhale, the energy flow from your sacral chakra to your Heart Chakra. Do this for a duration of seven breaths.

Repeat this exercise over and over to suit your need. After you do this exercise for the first time, you will notice a pleasant change in body, mind, and spirit. Continue peacefully. There are no limits to the positive changes in the work of the chakra.

Positive spiritual experiences and the ability to forgive lead to better physical health, while negative spiritual experiences are linked to worse physical and mental health for people, and love brings all this together.

Chakras provide the spiritual energy our bodies need to help them cope with daily anxiety. Chakra tuning allows you to understand yourself and the world around you more fully. The value of doing so is to keep your lives well balanced.

Think of the chakras as aspects of consciousness, as auras that are not like our corporal physical. They interact in the endocrine and nervous systems with our bodies. A specific part of our human anatomy is connected to each chakra.

If they are concentrated, the chakras give more concentration and energy to your mind and body. Proper synchronization allows the mind and body to function together. This makes us happy and calmer.

Why tune chakras?

Everything you need to self-tune your chakras, you already have inside. You don't need any special instrument or membership fees. You change your chakras to find harmony and re-energize yourself, which is the secret to excellent wellness.

Think of Chakras as vibrations that respond to color and sound. You will restore the chakras to their original beauty and strength by visualizing the colors and tones of each chakra. Therapeutic chakra music vibrates the seven chakras in perfect harmony. This balances mind and spirit in the whole body of healing, meditation, and relaxation.

Chakra meditation starts by sitting in a relaxed position with your spine straight. Then you want to concentrate on every part of your body, starting with your legs. When you do, that part of your body needs to relax and let the tension melt away.

The next phase in chakra meditation is to focus on breathing. Don't push it, but let the breathing be steady and strong. Your mind will most likely wander, just gently bring it back to your breath and keep your attention in every inhalation and exhalation you take. Visualize the oxygen that comes into your lungs and passes through the bloodstream. Visualize it by nourishing all the muscles, organs and cells of your body, and then see it by extracting the toxins from your body that you remove with each step.

Next in the meditation of the chakra, you want to visualize the beat of the heart and the perfect function of the body. See how all of the pieces work together in full harmony. See how the oxygen sustains all of these parts and the body as a whole. Be conscious that breathing is life-sustaining energy to the whole organism that you call your body.

Next, in chakra meditation, you can imagine a life-giving force that you're breathing in along with the air. See this energy as the hue of yellowish-orange. See the energy as it surrounds your whole body and infuse your aura. As this energy infuses the aura, imagine the aura becoming bigger, brighter and charged with this incredible energy. Do this phase slowly, let the aura grow brighter little by little, and keep the energy flowing in with each breath.

The next phase we want to do in the meditation of the chakra is to energize each individual chakra. Start with the root chakra at the bottom of the back. Picture a clockwise vortex of energy and the air with which you breathe activates this ripple and makes it stronger and brighter. First, we want to imagine another stream of energy coming out of the planet. It is the same life that gives energy and contributes to the spinning energy of the Root Chakra.

First, in the practice of the chakra, we want to step up to the Sacred Chakra. Then one by one: the Solar Plexus Chakra, the Heart Chakra, the Throat Chakra, the Brow Chakra, and later the Crown Chakra, infusing each with life-giving energy. Take your time with this and don't think about spending more time on one chakra if you need to. It is highly recommended that you always work from the bottom up and not skip around. Increasing chakra will affect the other chakras and energize the higher chakra until the lower chakra may have an adverse effect.

The last step in the meditation of the chakras is to visualize all the chakras at once to be fed by the energy coming in from the breath and up from the earth. Always remember to see the chakras and your aura get stronger, simpler, and super- charged with giving energy to this existence.

Now, we can open our eyes and relax with our eyes open for a few minutes. Pay attention to your body and how amazing and energized you feel right now. Seek to practice for 15-30 minutes every sitting. Enjoy, this is a very healthy, uplifting meditation on the chakra.

Using Our Chakras To Tweak Our Health And Happiness

1. Root Chakra (base of your spine, legs, blood, bones) – We're all about feeling rooted, healthy, and supported here. It's our survival instinct, our ability to feel at home in our body, our connection to our immediate family. Think about the basics: food, shelter and money. Many of the underlying physical

health problems include eating disorders, asthma, autoimmune diseases, and rectal cancer.

Modification tips for the Root Chakra:

Do you have an unfinished business with a family member? Write a letter to them, mail it to yourself (not to them unless you know the letter is going to do more good than harm), read it, and burn it.

Get "grounded," plant a garden, go for a walk, walk barefoot in the grass.

Eat root vegetables and add some more animal protein to your diet. Then thank the animals, the plants, the people who grow / farm for helping you.

2. Sacral Chakra (navel region, reproductive organs, kidney, bladder, lower back) – The second chakra is all about sex and creativity, personal ethics and morals, and interacting consciously with others outside our family unit. Some of the associated physical health issues include lower back pain, reproductive organ disease, bladder cancer, infertility problems, and kidney disease.

Modification tips for the Sacred Chakra:

Think about your relationship with power, sex, and money. Are you a little over-controlling? Or are you feeling guilty, shameful? Find the balance here.

Create a vision board for what you want.

Prepare your meal and share it with your friends.

You really have to interact with the flavors and textures of your food. Render a sensual feeling of eating.

3. Solar Plexus (digestion, gallbladder, liver, pancreas, adrenals) - This is all about self-esteem, confidence, self-care, and how we perceive ourselves in comparison to others. Are you worried that you would fail? This is a common weakness of the third chakra. Some of the physical health conditions related to the solar plexus include anemia,

ulcers, diabetes, digestive disorders, and liver disease.

Modifying tips for the third chakra:

Eat with your mind. Chew your food thoroughly.

Pamper yourself, take a long bath, or create a soothing ritual before bedtime.

Prepare your meal and share it with your friends. Meditate on respecting and appreciating who you are.

4. Heart Chakra (pulmonary, heart, circulatory system) - Here we are all about love, love without condition, forgiveness, compassion, acceptance of people who are different from us. An underactive heart chakra can manifest itself as feeling unloved, racist, and outwardly pursuing affection rather than cultivating self-love. Some Heart Chakra-related illnesses include heart disease, respiratory problems, breast cancer, and upper back pain.

Modification tips for the heart chakra:

Lead by example.

Eat more bitter greens (kale, watercress, arugula, bok choy). Keep a journal of appreciation.

5. Throat Chakra (thyroid, ears, arms, neck) – This is where we focus on our willingness to let go of material

ties or items that no longer serve us. This chakra connects us to our spirit, and it represents our ability to communicate effectively with others, our true voice. Some of the physical health issues related to the Throat Chakra include thyroid problems, chronic sore throat, esophageal cancer, and pain in the shoulder and neck.

Modifying tips for the Throat Chakra:

Sing, engage in drama (performance, not the kind of energy- sucking event) and write.

Meditate as you concentrate on your breathing. Express what you stand for.

6. Third eye (between eyebrows, pineal gland, eyes) - Do you ever get that "aha!" moment? This chakra is for intelligence, imagination, and dreaming. It's represented by light and our circadian rhythm. There are many emotional illnesses manifested here: obsessive-compulsive behavior blocked thinking, always relying on others for guidance, and poor self- awareness.

Modifying tips for the sixth chakra:

Tap on your intuition. Turn the electronics off and sit down in silence. Listen to your inner voice, please. Practice this every day for 20 minutes.

Eat seasonally and locally and use fresh herbs and spices to cook.

Reduce your intake of caffeine and alcohol.

7. Crown Chakra (top of the head, pituitary gland, cerebral cortex) – The seventh chakra is the furthest away from the physical body and material objects. It is our spirituality, our confidence in divine power, and from where we derive faith and hope. Emotional diseases of the Crown Chakra include feeling lost without purpose in life, schizophrenia, depression, and suicidal thoughts.

Modifying tips for the crown chakra:

Take the time to "clean up" your mind. Heck, you're not talking twice about washing your dirty clothes. Push out negative emotions and breathe into positive ones.

Practice your spirituality: church, synagogue, prayer, meditation, spells, whatever they may be.

Reflect on why you're so happy about your life.

Reason You Can't Clear Your Chakras

People who have studied spiritual healing and understand how strong and essential the chakras are generally searching for ways to begin clearing them. Sadly, many people are misguided to believe that they can clear their own chakras with meditation, crystals, colors, Reiki, or other forms of self-help. Unfortunately, it never works. It's difficult to clear up any stress without being mindful of what it is first and finding a way to get someone else to take it out of you. You need to work with a clear-sighted spiritual healer who can see what thoughts, memories, false perceptions, and old traumas you've had in your chakras and energy field. After you are told the exact events or emotions that block you and the truth can be confirmed, you can release it to a healer who can take him off your field and fill your spine with pure, highly vibrating energy. Working with a real clairvoyant does not just let you confirm and release exactly what's in your chakras, you also remove low vibration or evil forces from your chakras that cannot be handled in any other mode. The power of these evil parasite beings is the source of much of a person's suffering and misery. The difference is clear and amazing when removed, and even the unbelievers and skeptics are persuaded of that!

Many techniques, such as meditation, do not work to clear the chakras or eliminate entities. In reality, they can be dangerous if you've been tricked to open your chakras, or if you're suffering under the control of the force, as this opens your mind to it even more. Your chakras are like a faucet of water. When you force your chakras to open, it's like turning the hot water tap all the way. In a few minutes, you've drained all the hot water out of the tank, and you're not going to be able to refill it, so the water is running cold. Worse, having a chakra forced to open will unbalance it. There are many cases of anxiety when the chakra is too open. When the Heart Chakra is too open, codependent behavior can be seen. Like your pupils, your chakras react to situations and know how open the circumstances are. Anyone who tells you to force your chakras open as far as they go is completely uninformed and cannot "see" how this advice affects your energy being the way a true clairvoyant can.

Working with someone who "heals" crystal chakras can be just as dangerous. Many people who deal with crystals don't understand how healing works. They believe the stones are going to yield magical effects. They don't need to have any clear-sighted ability to do this, and they often don't know what they're doing. They don't know if the crystals they're using have a positive effect. They don't know where they're meant to be, so they can't see how the jumbling of different stones with different energies together impacts the energy field. They can't see how dangerous it is to put crystals on the chakras, either! In fact, I had customers who were coming with "burns" from misinformed "healers," who used a crystal laser wand on the chakra! This produces a powerful picture, just like a scar to clean up a few times before the chakra can work correctly. Many of my clients told me that after having had contact with crystal "healers," they had significant problems with their bodies and in their lives.

Reiki and other forms of energy therapy, where people seek to clear your chakras or push energy into you, isn't therapy at all, even though they call themselves "Masters." You are the source of the energy that blocks your chakras and your life. No one can go in and see something that another person has made. You're the only one that can do this on your own. This is because we live on the Free Will plane, where our own decisions decide our own experiences. It's a world of karma, and we're responsible for what we make. We must therefore all agree to release our own energy. All it does is 'dislocate' friction and barriers when someone uses reiki and drives energy towards them. It may seem to make a temporary difference, but it usually wears off quickly and can cause further problems as energy manifests itself in new ways. This also means that people who get attracted to a Reiki practitioner have to keep coming back on a regular to keep seeing the effects. Reiki cannot clear the energies of your chakras or heal them. After your energy (qi) has been released (by you), the only time that reiki can be used effectively is to fill in what was purged.

A lot of people are very impressed by the sound healing-a practice that involves a sound frequency like singing bowls or CDs. They tell me that they can feel something going on in their chakras and believe it works. Sadly, what they don't realize is that what they hear is the emotional vibration of the tone chakra, which causes the chakra to vibrate in response to the sound in which it resonates. It may be felt physically, but it does not indicate that the energy is released or that the chakra is healed or changed. Such clients go away amazed by the "healing" received because they could sense something going on, and then they're surprised when we clear up 90 minutes of old incidents, traumas, feelings, and malicious forces in their chakras afterward.

Since getting clarity with a clairvoyant spiritual chakra healer operating with

Free Will, most people can't believe how amazing they feel and how noticeable their findings are from other approaches. You will feel warm, fresh, satisfied, relaxed and some people will feel even youthful again! They start seeing changes in their thoughts and emotions and even how people respond to them. Sometimes they're able to see issues in their lives improve as they're able to manifest themselves better. You should find a genuine clairvoyant energetic chakra healer and witness the difference that real clearing should create. You'll be shocked how different you feel even after years of reiki, meditation, light and crystal healing, and a number of other techniques. You will also be shocked at the many things that you can confirm and know to be in your chakras, which the far-sighted man will find! Learn yourself and see how a complete healing system can make a difference in your life today!

Creating Through Chakras

If you don't think you're a creative artist, think again. You create your life every moment of every day. Where could you possibly be more imaginative than that?

You are experiencing a creative spiritual connection when you become so involved with whatever you create that the rest of the world is fading away. You're losing all track of time. You will still forget about the last time you eat. Inspiration appears to float to you and around you. So it is. inspiration is coming to you through your Crown Chakra.

You see, your chakras are more than just whirlpools of energy all over your body. In fact, they are a very sophisticated system for exchanging information in the form of energy. For example, visions are received in the Third Eye Chakra, inspiration is received through the Crown Chakra.

However, you can use your chakras to obtain energy from other people and your surroundings more than unconsciously. You can consciously use them for a variety of purposes, including for creation.

Use your chakras at any time during the creative process to enhance inspiration, passion, vision and more. You will find that the flow of the entire process will be much smoother and easier, from the beginning of the inspiration to the final manifestation. Be imaginative with the energy of your chakras and discover the difference that they can make.

The spiritual growth through the chakras

The imaginative life force sleeps inside each one of us like a coiled serpent, waiting to be unleashed to bring humanity to the next level. Ancient Tantric practices awaken this force, called kundalini, by using the body, the air, the sound, and the visualizations to speed up its path to the realization of God.

Men have three bodies: their bodies or their consciences, their astral bodies, and their causal bodies, their thoughts and feelings, their knowledge and wisdom. It's the root cause. The seven chakras serve as energy transformers for the three bodies/minds that each has specific functions. It purifies the body/mind with every chakra triggered, spiritualizing the subject and increasing consciousness. The energy progressively moves out of the darkness, the negative, the light, the good poles and the entire consciousness of the seventh chakra. The technique was related to western psychoanalysis.

FIRST CHAKRA

The Muladhara Chakra, on the coccyx, is a negative axis. You're bonded to setting values at this level. Safety and self- preservation are the main themes. Primitive energies, such as fear, struggle and flight, are the prevalent response to physical or psychological attacks or injuries. You are experiencing intense global fear causing extinction. This chakra is linked to anxiety, addiction and extreme illness, which can contribute to violence towards others. Such concerns are more deeply rooted in the average person, but they can still affect one's life. Where these impulses are disowned, they are protruded to be hurtful to others. Growth begins as these fears become integrated, conscious, and transformed. When unconscious impulses or memories are brought to consciousness, more energy is made accessible for higher functioning. When the sleeping serpent slowly wakes up and rises, you may begin to feel the sensations of floating, bliss, tingling and warmth at the base of your spine. Clairvoyance or clairaudience may appear.

SECOND CHAKRA

The second, Svadhisthana, is below the naval level and above the genitals.

Your senses and nervous system are becoming more sensitive, affecting you both physically and emotionally. The emphasis is more on sexual and sensual gratification than on protective self-protection. There is therefore greater interaction with others, albeit as sexual objects, and a wider range of emotions, even though you are still controlled by unconscious impulses and appetites. Such procreative energies are very strong, and if they are not articulated, sublimated or guided upward, they can be mentally and physically very uncomfortable. Meditation and Tantric sexual practices provide tools for channeling kundalini to higher centers.

This chakra is widely considered the seat of the unconscious, and once opened, you may be overwhelmed by strong, sometimes conflicting emotions. All your past conditioning and patterns are revealed and acted upon, and if you do not analyze or work through increasing consciousness, the kundalini will arise. Higher transpersonal levels of conscious awareness can only be archived after you are personal subconscious has been successfully explored and integrated. There are warnings that unless you have enough ego strength, character, and faith in God. The energies you release may cause great harm to the individual, from improper sexual or romantic attachments to mental breakdown. This chakra awakens knowledge of the astral body and increased intuition. Prophetic visions and telepathic experiences can also take place.

THIRD CHAKRA

The third one, Manipura, is close in proxemics with the solar plexus. The problem here revolves around control and power and the need to meet your personal needs in the world. The goal is to assert yourself effectively in the world without manipulating, exploiting or subjugating others. As Manipura awakens, you become conscious of your spirit, gain control over your emotions, and thus begin to exercise power beyond your own karma. Some traditions find this to be the beginning of spiritual development, because of the propensity for kundalini to descend if you have not overcome the trials of the second chakra. You can also encounter digestive issues here while the body is being cleaned. There is a higher ESP capability.

FOURTH CHAKRA

The fourth, Anahata or the heart chakra, is in the center of the nipples. When Anahata is fully awoken, you are separated from your feelings and transcended karma. Feelings are less contaminated with needs and addictions. You are aware of your feelings and karmic patterns, but you can exercise your free will to fulfill your wishes. Now the soul can guide your choices and actions more fully. Having tamed basic survival instincts and needs (in the first three chakras), there is sufficient energy to concentrate on self-realization. This chakra is therefore considered to be the intersection between the earthly and the divine, as well as the left (yin) and the right (yang). This is represented by the sign of the cross and also by the six-pointed star consisting of two triangles. Your mind is gradually in the spirit realm.

In the heart area, you may feel stabbing pain. Eventually, this is followed by a surrender of the fight for power and a desire to be more and more guided by the spirit. In the Jungian context, there is a greater balance and interaction between the ego and the self. As a result, there is less internal conflict and more harmony with yourself and others, as well as less projection and division of good and bad. As you become more integrated and cohesive, there is less attachment and demand for others and greater care, responsiveness and respect for them. You can give without the need to receive or manipulate others for personal gratification. A positive attitude to life develops, and this is considered important to the preservation of the evolution of Kundalini. Psychokinetic and healing forces emerge, and synchronicity and wishful fulfillment begin to take place.

FIFTH CHAKRA

The fourth, Vishuddhi, is in the throat and the thyroid gland. Vishuddhi is linked to soulful expression and creativity. It includes the ability to set the ego aside and allow higher self or creative intelligence to be expressed verbally and artistically. Similarly, the throat chakra controls the ability to receive nourishment from others and from the divine. Gradually, you develop a sense of trust and security, realizing that infinite sustenance originates from the inner transpersonal source. When you reach out to the unknown and trusting spirit to evolve and develop, you cultivate yourself in the act of creation. You begin to function with greater detachment in the world, increasingly linked to the spiritual realm.

It is also said that this core governs our sense of time and space, whether we feel time passing slowly or rapidly, influencing the rhythm of our lives. Hearing may sharpen, and telepathic powers may be eventually created.

SIXTH CHAKRA

The sixth chakra is called Ajna, is between the eyebrows near the pineal gland and the pituitary gland. The pineal gland is associated with vision and light. You can see light around the forehead when this chakra is triggered. Intuition and insight are heightened. You can contact your higher wisdom or your inner guru. The inner vision obtained brings you beyond the physical dimension and beyond the limitation of time, space and causality. You feel connected to nature and to the entire universe. This experience reflects the coming together of two kinds of knowledge — feeling and intellectual. The two, left and right, feminine and masculine nadis or channels, join the Ajna Chakra, symbolized by the caduceus.

SEVENTH CHAKRA

The seventh, Sahasrara, is the positive pole at the top of the head. When the kundalini activates this chakra, the Brahman Gate opens and the divine energy enters, symbolized by the crown, halo or light. At first, you feel headaches and brief moments of samadhi; this further stimulates all the other chakras. With practice, length and effects are increasing. When you are fully active, duality disappears, and you achieve cosmic consciousness, samadhi, or enlightenment. God is perceived as a state of being; there are no longer unconscious feelings or thoughts, nor is there a distinction between self and the understanding of feeling or thinking. You become pure consciousness and have a profound understanding of yourself and the true nature of all things and all dimensions.

Sahasrara is in a "soft place," which closes down gradually after the spirit comes in, then opens again to leave when she dies. Adepts can prepare themselves for their time of death when their mind will forever leave their body. In order to protect the region, the Orthodox Jews wear a skull cap while some monks shave their heads.

There are other rituals for the awakening of the chakras. One strategy is to concentrate on each chakra when looking at the top of the nose. Another custom is to imagine the associated color at each chakra and to sing the correct mantra.

The order that the chakras are awakening varies with the karma and nature of each person. Many suffer from this powerful force, physically and psychologically, are unable to live a normal life and are never given the desired benefits, so it is very necessary to learn and to avoid hastening the cycle with an experienced instructor.

CHAPTER FOUR

Empowering And Opening Our Chakras To Improve Ourselves

What do I feel when they're out of balance? If your chakras are out of control, you might feel like you're in a mess, as if your life has been held back, but you don't know why. You may feel less than optimal, less energetic and less healthy. A chakra that may be out of control can be mirrored in your life in the areas of your body where it is located. For example, if you are a person who has regular sore throats, it may be that your Throat Chakra is not healthy or does not work at its highest potential. Applying healing techniques that are directly related to the Throat Chakra would be beneficial. (Note: it is not recommended that you rely solely on balancing chakras to alleviate a medical condition; it is always appreciated that you consult with your medical practitioner for chronic conditions.)

How Chakra Impairment Can Affect Life

There are varieties of beliefs about how many chakras are kept within the body and which the primary ones are. Think of the "chakra" as the "energy center;" there are many energy centers within the body, such as the palms of our hands. The seven major chakras that protrude from the base of the spine to the top of the head are most known in today's culture. This is the system that I use for most of the work I do.

This does not mean that the other chakra systems are not as valid or as vital as the seven-chakra system. Each system is essential in its own way; however, in terms of the energies that we deal with on a regular basis in the physical realm, it is most productive to concentrate first on the seven major chakras.

Like various systems in the body, one's chakra systems may become unbalanced. Such imbalances could have been harmful. Ideally, the energy of our chakras should work together at all times to manifest our desires in our physical life.

Unfortunately, many of us also concentrate too much energy on one specific area of life, and because "energy flows where attention is focused," the effect could be too many energies flow through that chakra and into the area of our lives.

Unfortunately, so many of us still concentrate on a specific region of our lives, so that too much energy will flow into that chakra and therefore into the field of our lives, as "energetic flows where attention goes. "For instance, the seventh chakra, also known as the Crown Chakra, is the home of spiritual energy and its place in our lives. And the first chakra, or Root Chakra, focuses on basic physicality and survival in our everyday lives. Many that tend to concentrate too much attention on spirituality rather than day-to-day affairs can potentially create a chakra imbalance: too much attention flowing into and out of the seventh chakra and not enough into the first chakra.

You may wonder what harm this imbalance can do. The first chakra has a lot to do with basic needs and concerns like food, paying bills, housing, and even the level at which you can manifest your needs and desires in your life. If we spend too little attention on the first chakra, we can find that we lose track of expenses, money doesn't come in as it used to, or maybe the house is a mess — all items that have a huge effect on our performance in our everyday lives.

There are many ways to ensure balance in the chakras, from visualizations and meditations that you can find on the internet to just wearing colors that equate to a specific chakra. All of these can be true and efficient ways of managing them, but clearing practice is also extremely successful in calming the chakras.

Why do I have to balance my chakras?

When your chakras are balanced, you may feel mentally clearer, more energetic, more creative, and healthier. The body is a wonderful healer if you're going to give it the best tools to work with. Balancing the chakras is one way to give it the tools you need. Think of when you're hungry, your body can't make food of its own, but it needs help from you. Give your body what it needs to start the healing process by balancing the "food" of your chakras.

How do I balance my chakras?

There are many therapies ranging from Reiki, massage, meditation, essential oils, sound and vibration therapy to chakra balancing. The purpose of balancing the chakra, otherwise known as waking the chakra, is to balance the energy of the body. Your emotions live and work as much as your physical body does. If one aspect is damaged or blocked, it can also affect your emotional health. Chakras are focal points for your energies, starting at your head and going down your spine.

Your chakras are intertwined, so if one of them is blocked, cascading effects can be extremely damaging. Think of your physical body as computer hardware; it's a functional machine that runs as long as it's maintained and has power (such as food, drink, etc.). Without the proper software, a computer cannot function. Your chakras work like computer software, harnessing their power for specific purposes. Like a computer, your energy system can pick up harmful energies. Chakra balancing works in the same way as a virus detection program, cleaning the system to avoid long-term damage.

There are a number of recommended techniques for chakra balancing.

Hands-on approach is a traditional approach to balancing chakras. It requires a detailed understanding of how the chakras relate to each other, so it is often recommended that you go to a professional.

Emotional Freedom Technique (EFT) involves taping key energy points on your body and reciting affirmations and resolutions.

Gemstones are also used to clean and trigger chakras. You place specific stones on each of them, and you sing special mantras, known as seed sounds,

Meditation is the easiest and most powerful process. It involves being in a relaxed physical state while focusing on a particular chakra.

Balanced chakras will make it easier for you to relate to goals that feel right for you on a profoundly emotional level.

Chakra Stones are a specific chakra balancing system. You place a specific stone (each chakra has one) on a chakra, and you meditate.

Chakra balancing with Ho'oponopono brainwave training will balance, cleanse, and activate your vortex chakras as you ask the Divine to release and dissolve blocks into white light.

Brainwave training is a vehicle that enhances Ho'oponopono's spiritual process. This scientifically proven technology changes the brain's frequency by introducing specific sound patterns in a repetitive and rhythmic way that the brain then mimics. Access to various individual chakra frequency can be reached quickly and easily, and when combined with the Ho'oponopono mantra, anything that hinders their full power potential will be cleaned and dissolved.

If your chakras are unbalanced or closed, you cannot integrate the level of consciousness that each chakra represents. Long holding negative states triggered by past emotional responses and thought patterns can block a chakra and can have a great effect on your physical, mental, emotional, and spiritual health.

Your life is going to be out of balance.

Chakras function as gates for light energy, — a vital energy for the life force entering the physical body — while simultaneously serving as a starting point for less frequency energies to return to the white light for transmutation in the United Area of Consciousness.

Asking the Divine, when every chakra is triggered by Ho'oponopono mantra, to be in direct communication with All That Is, removes, purifies and releases the negative, lower frequency gathered into the white light of the One Consciousness region.

Each of the seven major chakras is a level of awareness or a state of growth. When they are open and balanced, they form an integrated system that relies on each other for optimal health. All chakras are affected by blocking in one chakra.

The Importance of each Chakra Being Balanced Root Chakra

- Represents your foundation, your movement, your energy and survival, and your feeling of being grounded. This chakra binds you to the rhythms and patterns of nature.

- Influences your finances and all the things that have to do with survival.

- When unbalanced, it affects your liver and your adrenals, your back, your hip and your stability, and may interfere with your well-being.

Sacred Chakra

- Reflects your desire to embrace others, your new experience, and your relation to others.

- Gives you a feeling of wealth, intimacy, enjoyment and well-being.

- When unbalanced, problems arise in the kidneys, large and small intestines, pancreas, spleen, groin, prostrate and uterus. Your desire to enjoy sex can be hampered.

Solar Plexus Chakra

- Represents your ability to be confident and to be in control.

- Personal concern.

- Self-worth, self-esteem and self-confidence.

- When unbalanced, the immune system is affected, and you are prone to ulcers, hypoglycemia and stress- related illnesses. An impaired Solar Plexus can manifest as insecurities and personal concerns.

Heart Chakra

- It reflects the willingness to love, care and share.

- When unbalanced, there could be issues with the heart, high blood pressure, claustrophobia, feeling unfulfilled, helpless, constrained, and possessive or obsessive. An inhibited Heart Chakra may have you constantly looking for reassurance because of a lack of self-worth.

Throat Chakra

- It represents your ability to communicate.

- Contact and self-expression.

- When unbalanced, it causes issues with the mouth, head, spine, and thyroid. You have trouble expressing yourself, or you don't understand what you're communicating.

Third Eye Chakra

- Reflects your desire to see a broader picture and your imagination.

- Intuition, creativity, knowledge, understanding, dream, belief.

- When you are unbalanced, your mind is unclear, your thoughts are erratic, your intuition is blocked, and you have headaches and severe nightmares.

Crown Chakra

- Represents the highest Chakra and the desire to be fully connected with the Divine Intellect, the relation of your soul and feeling totally complete.

- Your link with the Spirit.

- When you are unbalanced, you feel alone and not connected to someone or something.

When you use the Ho'oponopono mantra when exercising your brain with brain-wave meditation, any blockage will be removed and equilibrium restored so that life-force energy can flow freely both up and down your body, linking all the chakras, each spinning at the same speed.

Ho'oponopono is a great cleaning practice because you don't need to know why your chakra may be unbalanced in order to release the blockages. Brainwave training will provide the ideal frequency to open each chakra for direct cleaning and balancing. Clearing and balancing each of your chakras will make it possible for you to live your best life. Take advantage of the technology, brainwave training, which can easily access and maintain the frequency needed to activate the chakras.

The Root Chakra Balancing and Healing

The Root Chakra, also known as the first chakra or the physical chakra, represents our connection to the Earth. This is situated at the end of the spinal cord, the tail bone, and it regulates the growth of bones and muscle strength. The physical chakra represents our physicality, vitality, and instincts of survival. It's related to our nose and our legs. The nose represents our animal instincts and the most primitive way to feel good and bad, and the feet are the root that holds us to Earth.

Each chakra represents a specific color of the rainbow; for the first chakra, the color is red, and the color is related to wealth and abundance. The actual chakra is also the center of manifestation, and the fulfillment of all our actual wants and needs depends on the balance of this chakra.

Physical chakras develop during the pregnancy phase of the mother until the first year of age of the infant; this is the stage where the need for safety and protection is greatest. It is therefore important to keep the child safe and make him or her feel loved at this stage in order for the first chakra to develop well.

Pregnancy problems, child abuse, and neglect of the mother are some of the causes of distress in the first chakra. Since this chakra also represents physicality, trauma and abuse experienced by a person, it also disrupts the flow of energy in the physical chakra, as these experiences make us feel lost and unsafe.

The physical pleasures that we feel from a happy and open first chakra are counteracted by terror, anxiety and uncertainty as we lose our grip on Earth. Obesity is a common symptom experienced by those with an imbalanced first chakra.

When we feel like we've lost our grip on life, the usual answer is to eat to try and regain equilibrium or to deprive ourselves of food because we want to drown in self-pity. Insecurity is also a common symptom of a disturbed first chakra. Insecurity can also be expressed by greed, material addiction, envy, and fear of drastic change. It may also results in a loss of relationship with friends and family and a lack of financial and material abundance.

Physical chakra is essential for balancing our manifestations. It is the chakra that is responsible for the success of all our physical and human needs. The first chakra is also responsible for our basic survival instincts, the need for health, physical balance, and vitality. These qualities benefit greatly from a safe and open first chakra.

When all is well in the first chakra, it means that our body remains well-rooted on Earth and results in an increase in self- esteem and a better self-image, and it also represents a time when we feel most confident about our overall position in life. A happy first chakra also leads to an increase in our relationship with people who matter to us because all kinds of anxiety and fear decreases when the first chakra is healthy and available.

The chakra system functions as one unit so that when one of the chakras is disturbed, the entire system is affected as well. This explains the importance of keeping the first chakra open and balanced while maintaining the general well-being of life.

Rebalancing and Healing The First Chakra

As well as causing particular complications on its own, the imbalanced Root Chakra may also have a knock-on impact on the body's entire energy system, contributing to more adverse effects. It is, therefore, necessary to correct chakra imbalances when they occur, and also to take steps to ensure that a balanced structure remains in place.

Crystals can be useful in preserving and achieving a chakra balance, and in the case of Root Chakras, red-colored stones such as garnet, red jasper, rhodochrosite and rubies may be beneficial, and even gray or black-colored stones such as hematite and black opal.

Meditation is also very useful for Root Chakra tuning, particularly if you use a brainwave meditation recording containing the sounds of the right frequencies to help this chakra return to alignment.

In case you're not already familiar with this, brainwave entrainment recordings contain rapidly repeated sounds of different frequencies. These may be used for reaching a number of relatively simple mental states and can include a particular frequency associated with a safe chakra function in the case of chakra healing. By listening to a recording every day, a well-tuned chakra system should be easier to restore and maintain.

The Second Chakra of Balance and Healing

The sacral chakra is associated with the orange color and is symbolized by a six-petal lotus flower. It refers to the regulation of the reproductive and urinary systems, as well as the adrenal glands and other digestive functions. At the mental and emotional level, this second chakra is linked to creativity, imagination and sexuality. The imbalances in the second chakra may manifest as reproductive problems, problems with the kidneys and the urinary system, jealousy and addictive behavior.

Balancing The Sacral Chakra

Unlike other chakras in the system, the second chakra can be returned to equilibrium by a number of approaches, including the use of crystals and meditation. Placing orange gemstones such as citrine or orange aventurine in the lower abdominal region when meditating can have a beneficial effect on this chakra. Even if you don't want to use crystals, meditation alone can be very effective, particularly if you use a brainwave meditation recording specifically designed to rebalance the second chakra.

If you're not already familiar with this, brainwave meditation involves listening to repetitive sounds of specific frequencies. Such sounds can directly affect the brain, making it easier to experience a range of altered states. In the case of chakra meditation, such recording may also include sounds of frequencies corresponding to those associated with healthy chakra function (as with all other parts of the physical and energetic body, the chakras are essentially vibrational in nature and are therefore susceptible to influence by other vibrational forces such as sound).

When you plan to use brainwave recording to align your chakra, make sure you set aside some time to listen regularly every day. Although some people get great results the first time they try, it's more normal to get the best results with regular practice than with anything else.

The flow of energy in this chakra can be described as something like the coherent forces of attraction that govern chemical bonding. The Sacred Chakra, therefore, is concerned with our concept of attraction and the development of our relationships with ourselves and others.

This is where we develop flexibility and fluidity as the second chakra is generally responsible for fluids in the body, especially lymphatic system fluids and synovial fluids in the joints. The color of the rainbow associated with the second chakra is the color orange, and the common symbol is the rising moon, all of which reflect our emotions and our relationships with others. The moon represents the light that comes from the sun just as people also mirror and share the energies and experiences of each other.

The chakra system is the energy center of our body that regulates our overall well-being. It acts as a single entity, and as a result, even if only one chakra is blocked or unbalanced, the entire chakra system is affected. This means the importance of keeping each chakra open and balanced. An open chakra leads to a balanced life and an overall sense of well-being.

If the second chakra is not accessible, or if the energy that flows out of it is not in harmony with that of the other chakras, one can experience a massive burst of emotion and an obsession with sexual thoughts. A blocked Sacral Chakra can also lead to lack of creativity, detachment from others, jealousy, guilt, oversensitivity, emotional dependence, and a poor understanding of boundaries and limits.

When our second chakra is not kept open, we usually lose our attachment to our relatives and friends, and we return to keeping everything to ourselves. However, the second chakra is also linked to our self-esteem, and thus a significant imbalance and blockade of the second chakra may lead to self-denial and rejection of something that makes us feel good.

Physical manifestations of imbalanced second chakra include chronic lower back pain, adrenal exhaustion, sexually transmitted diseases, and infertility. In the worst-case scenario, a blocked second chakra leads to the development of eating disorders, such as anorexia, and even manic depression.

To keep the second chakra open and healthy, we can focus on some yoga exercises, color therapy, sound therapy, and energy healing, among others. Some of the best ways to keep the second chakra safe is by wearing orange-colored clothing and having orange ornaments and decorations at home and at work.

One of the major advantages of having an open second chakra is having a high sense of physical pleasure, emotional satisfaction, and creative expression. Having an open chakra allows for an open and honest relationship with the people we love. In general, it inspires a great passion for life, marriage, sex and good food.

Third Chakra Balancing and Healing

The third chakra is associated with the yellow and is represented by a 10-petalled lotus flower. As far as physical functioning is concerned, it is related to the functioning of the digestive system and a mental and emotional level; it is correlated with personal strength, ego and self-esteem and individual development. Strong instinct or intuition is also related to this chakra. Solar Plexus imbalances in the chakra can manifest as digestive problems with the liver and pancreas, and feelings of low self-esteem and lack of self-confidence.

Dealing with Imbalances

Crystal healing can be an effective way of rebalancing the chakras, and for the third chakra, by using yellow or brown colored stones, such as the tiger's eye, the amber and the yellow tape, which can be placed over the solar plexus area. The third chakra may also benefit from the use of the brainwave training meditation setting, which includes frequencies explicitly designed to target this chakra.

In case you're unfamiliar with brainwave processing, it basically involves listening to a recording that contains fast- repeating sounds of specific frequencies. The chosen frequencies will depend on the result you are trying to achieve. In the case of the rebalancing of the chakra, the recording should contain the frequencies associated with the functioning of the healthy chakra.

Brainwave training also makes it easier to achieve a meditative state, which makes it particularly useful for those who want to take proper advantage of chakra meditation, but have difficulties relaxing deeply and staying focused.

Therefore, keeping the chakra open increases our self- confidence and guides us on how we discover and use our innate strengths and abilities. Yellow is the color of the rainbow that is associated with this chakra; it is the color of fire or the light. The sun is a universal source of energy, and it is also a source of energy for the chakra. The third chakra regulates digestion and metabolism.

The chakra system is a single entity; thus, if you want to keep it running smoothly, you need to make sure that it stays accessible and balanced. It is also important to remember that a specific aspect of human life is regulated by each chakra. However, once a single chakra is disrupted, the entire system will be affected and, as a result, our entire well-being will be jeopardized.

When the third chakra is interrupted, we feel either a lack of or overflowing energy. When there's too much pressure on the third chakra, our power quest normally goes into overdrive. It's the power we want with the third chakra, and while we're on the way to achieving it, maybe we're going overboard and getting into confrontations with others.

Other emotional expressions may include hate, rage, greed, misuse of power, personal dominance, and failure to acknowledge one's own faults. On the other hand, when the third chakra is blocked, it results in a lack of self-confidence, uncertainty in claiming personal strength, a feeling of losing control of one's own life, and depression. Physical manifestations include kidney stones, gallstones, or liver stones.

The importance of keeping the third chakra open and balanced is inevitable to maintain order in our lives. An open third chakra will lead to a feeling of complete control over one's life. It also gives you a sense of self-direction; of knowing what you want, and, more importantly, of knowing that you can get it.

The emotional benefits of an open chakra include cheerfulness, active feeling, high self-respect, creativity, happiness, risk-taking, and a strong sense of personal power. A happy and open Solar Plexus Chakra is what keeps us in a high mood, and that's why we're always going to achieve our goals. If we keep this chakra open and safe, we will feel a certain kind of fulfillment that is the product of acquired control, personal energy, and achievement.

Fourth Chakra Balancing and Healing

The fourth chakra is located behind the bone of the breast, at the level of the heart; therefore, it is also called the Heart Chakra. It is represented by a green color and a traditional 12- petaled lotus. The Heart Chakra is the core of everything. It is the center of love, compassion, and spirituality, and it dictates how we feel love for ourselves and how we share love with others. It is also the focal point of our entire life because it reflects the inner equilibrium and the strongest chakra in our hearts. In the chakra network, the fourth chakra is also the nucleus that binds our minds and souls. The lower chakras are our physical existence, while the upper chakras are our spiritual existence. Being in the middle, the fourth chakra is the balance between the two.

If the fourth chakra is blocked or unbalanced, it results in an overall disturbance of the chakra system. In particular, an imbalanced fourth chakra would often result in fear of intimacy and love, and one would tend to choose to run away from these emotions. If your fourth chakra is blocked, you might be able to cut off all your ties to the outside, which can make you very cynical and skeptical of all. As your heart becomes more closed, you will also become more isolated from the world. Physical symptoms would include low blood pressure, bronchitis, asthma, and other lung problems.

Some people have an over-open Heart Chakra. Some symptoms of an over-open chakra include heart disease and high blood pressure. Emotionally, an excessively open chakra will trigger too much reliance on the love of others that you fail to value yourself. This lets you live by the grace of the love and affection of others. It also results in jealousy and over- empathy. If you have an overly open Heart Chakra, you appear to drown in self-pity.

Keeping the fourth chakra open is essential to our overall well- being. The Heart Chakra is known as the center of self-healing and detoxification, keeping it healthy and open would greatly influence our trust and our ability to love ourselves. A happy and open Heart Chakra will contribute to a positive overall outlook in life. It helps you to see the beauty of the world, the beauty of others, and, of course, your own beauty. Getting an open chakra would also mean that you are able to forgive and you are very forgiving of other people's ways.

In the Hindu scriptures, the fourth chakra is known as the Sanskrit word "Anaharata," which means "unhappy." The Sanskrit term is the structure of the fourth chakra. When our hearts are broken, it causes a deep heart scar in our aura. The fourth chakra removes these scars and, as a result, it also removes the pain that created these scars, but under the pain, the heart heals and recovers its fullness and development.

Throat Chakra Balancing and Healing

The Throat Chakra, for the fifth chakra, is located in the neck area. In this section, we will look at its characteristics, the problems that may be caused by an imbalanced Throat Chakra, and the method you can use to stimulate and rebalance it at home.

What's the Throat Chakra?

Chakras are energy vortexes that play a key role in maintaining the health and integrity of your mind-body system, as well as connecting you with greater energy of the universe. The Throat Chakra is also known by the Sanskrit name 'vishuddha' and is one of the seven main chakras found in a line extending from the base of the spine to the crown of the head.

Fifth Chakra Characteristics

All chakras are associated with particular colors, energetic frequencies, areas of the body and other characteristics. The Throat Chakra is related to the color blue and the general qualities of self-expression, effective communication and intuitive guidance. As far as the physical body system is concerned, this chakra is associated with the neck, mouth, arms, hands and thyroid gland.

Throat chakra blockages can manifest as problems in these areas of the body, as well as communication problems with both others and/or your inner self.

Healing The Throat Chakra

If this chakra (or any chakra for that matter) becomes unbalanced, it is important to sort it out, as one chakra that is unbalanced can have a knock-on effect on the other chakras, as well as on your energy system as a whole.

One choice for healing the Throat Chakra is to visit an energy healer who may be able to intuitively sense and relax the chakra back to its optimum functioning. However, this is not a realistic choice for many people, and it can be difficult, in any case, to find a suitably experienced person who really knows what they are doing.

Remember, no one else is going to be as tuned to your chakra and energy system as you are, so you may find it easier to tune your Throat Chakra at home. Various chakra tuning techniques are available, such as the use of crystals and color healing. However, a chakra-balancing brainwave training recording is probably the simplest method.

A good recording of this type includes sounds of specific frequencies that have been specially chosen to stimulate the chakra in question and to bring it back into balance. You don't need to be a veteran meditator to use brainwave therapy, either, since the learning itself can help direct the brain into a profoundly relaxed and concentrated state. This makes it easier for those of us with "monkey minds" to enjoy the benefits of meditation without spending years of school.

When using a meditation recording for your Throat Chakra, it would normally be beneficial to listen regularly until you get the results you're looking for, and then revisit the recording periodically to give your chakras a tune-up as needed.

Look at our opinion as being as important as breathing air. Also, air is necessary to be alive; just as it is vital to live across our point in front of others. When we speak, our words convey our feelings to others. Our choice of words and the style of delivering them make people aware of our mood at a given time. For example, if someone wants to express love to the other person, he/she is likely to say "I love you" in a calm and soothing manner. Similarly, if someone is angry, he's going to choose harsh words to spread his point in a loud and screaming manner. All these mannerisms of speech and the way in which they are delivered are all controlled by the fifth chakra.

Now that we are aware of the value of the Throat Chakra, it would be a joy for us to come across the riches that it awards us. For a good Throat Chakra, we are able to interact and convey our thoughts in a better way. Communication involves not only talking but also listening to what others have to say. This operates in a two-way mode of transport. If one side is unanswered or blocked, it is the result of a blocked chakra. "I speak and I am heard" is the slogan that makes us live by this chakra. In addition, this chakra is also linked to our creativity. Improve communication, improve creativity.

In other words, we can only climb the ladder of success if we are clear about our desires and make others realize that. We are blessed with self-expression, free will and the eloquence of a healthy Throat Chakra.

Conversely, there are many factors that are working their way to block the pace of the Throat Chakra. This chakra is about spiritual truth as well as about speaking our own truth. So lies, half-truths, cheating, and other unfair means credit for chakra imbalance. Expressing excessive criticism and authoritarianism also poses problems for the chakra, which can lead to various tribulations such as gossip, addiction, voice domination and interruption. Although the energy in the chakra is low, it results in shyness, inconsistency, introversion and unreliability. It is therefore very important to ensure the good health of this chakra. Other than that, indigo-colored objects also tend to heal chakras like indigo-colored t-shirts or going by the sea.

All the chakras have their own significance in our lives. Unlike the rest of us, the Throat Chakra stands as one for which our chances of survival are slim.

The Sixth Chakra Balancing and Healing

Each chakra is connected and linked to a particular color, and in this case, the color is indigo. The Brow Chakra is strongly associated with intuition, and when it is well regulated, you will benefit from a consistent flow of inner wisdom and insight. It is also linked to the health of the head, including the eyes, ears and nose.

Keeping The Sixth Chakra in Balance

Chakras can even become imbalanced as a result of various causes, including the stressful lifestyles that so many people are living today. Such imbalances can manifest in a variety of ways, and in the case of the Third Eye Chakra, you may experience symptoms such as head problems, eyes, ears, etc., as well as a sense of confusion, mental concern, and learning difficulties.

As with other chakras, the use of crystals may be beneficial in restoring balance. The use of blue-colored gemstones such as sodalite or lapis lazuli may be beneficial for the brow chakra.

In addition, meditation is one of the most powerful ways to rebalance the sixth chakra, particularly if you use a brainwave training recording designed for this purpose. In case you're not familiar with it, brainwave training basically involves listening to the sounds of specific frequencies, with the frequencies in question depending on what the recording is intended to accomplish. This is great for people who are not trained meditators, and who may find it difficult to remain focused on traditional guided meditation techniques.

The Seventh Chakra of Balancing and Healing

This chakra is also known as "thousand-petalled lotus" and "Sahasrara" in traditional Sanskrit terms. It is associated with the colors white and purple and connects the individual with the larger spiritual self. A balanced seventh chakra fosters a sense of spiritual harmony and peace, as well as a strong sense of intuition. This is aligned with the top of the head region and the pineal gland in terms of its effect on the human body.

The imbalances in the Crown Chakra frequently manifest themselves as depression, apathetic behavior, and a sense of social alienation and inability to communicate with others.

Balancing the Crown Chakra

The seventh chakra can be rebalanced using a variety of methods, such as crystal healing. It is especially sensitive to diamonds, while clear crystal quartz often works very well, and can either be put in the crown region as part of a crystal healing session.

The use of meditation on the Crown Chakra can also be very beneficial. Traditional chakra meditation often involves the use of guided imagery, although modern technology has made it more efficient and easier to use for those who are not used to meditation, thanks to brainwave training.

If you use a brainwave training recording to tune the Crown Chakra, you will hear sounds of certain frequencies that have been found to have a direct and beneficial effect on this energy center. Like every other part of the mind-body complex, each chakra is associated with a specific frequency when it operates optimally, and exposure to the sound of the correct frequencies can help bring the chakra into balance with relatively little effort on your part.

To use this method, you should be prepared to set aside some time every day to listen to your recording in a quiet place where you won't be disturbed. Although a lot of people get great results right away, this isn't always the case, so it's important to be consistent and listen regularly. With some time and daily usage, a chakra-balancing meditation session can have a very beneficial effect on the wellbeing of your Crown Chakra.

Nowadays, many people are suffering from a lifestyle-related problem that most of them are not even aware of, and that is imbalanced chakras. A balanced chakra system is vital if you want to be as healthy as possible at the physical, mental, emotional and spiritual level, and long-term chakra blockages can lead to physical illness and other problems. In this book, we'll take a look at one of the best methods of clearing your chakras and rebalancing your chakra system from the comfort and privacy of your home.

Chakras are energy vortexes, which are located in different parts of the body. Although in total there are thousands of chakras, the primary chakra system consists of only seven.

They are positioned in a rough line from just below the chest to the top of the head. When these primary chakras are unbalanced, they have a knock-on impact on the rest of your body, and one unbalanced chakra can also cause problems with others.

Growing chakra vibrates at a different frequency when it operates properly, and negative lifestyle influences can contribute to any chakra slowing down or accelerating. Chakra blockages can manifest in a variety of ways, depending on the chakra that is affected, and the degree to which it is out of the way. For example, you may experience physical symptoms such as pain or numbness, obstructed creativity and emotions, or feel disconnected from your spiritual source. In order to remedy such symptoms, the chakra must be unblocked and brought back into balance with the rest of the system. After this is done, your energy can flow again freely.

Various methods of clearing the chakra are in use, and some people prefer to visit energy healers who can conduct work on calming the chakra. Such people may be able to intuitively perceive blockages in others' chakra systems, and such energy work can be effective. Nevertheless, finding an effective healer can be difficult, particularly if you don't live in an urban area, and sessions can also be costly. Also, there's always a danger posed by charlatans who have no expertise in this area, but who are happy to take your money anyway.

Luckily, it's possible to clear your own chakras, and it can actually be a good idea to do so because even the best energy practitioner will not be as close to your own energy system as you are. In other words, you should clear your chakras from the inside out, and this process is made simpler if you use a brainwave training recording tailored for this purpose.

Such recording features specific frequency sounds and will help you to become deeply relaxed and focused (something that most people who are not trained meditators have difficulty with during conventional meditation). Good recording will also include frequencies that have been found to stimulate the chakras, help in the clearing and rebalancing process.

When you use such a recording, you'll need to find a quiet spot to listen, where you're physically relaxed and you're not going to be interrupted. You should also listen to the recording each day (or as directed) in the beginning, and after you get the results you want, it's still a good idea to use the recording periodically, to give your chakra system a regular tune-up, and to prevent it from getting out of balance again.

Using A Chakra Meditation for Chakra Tuning

Unfortunately, chakras may become imbalanced due to various lifestyle causes, such as negative emotions, stress, etc. Such imbalanced chakras can rotate more slowly or quickly than normal, and instead of being a harmonious part of the body's energy system, they begin to have a destructive impact. If left unchecked, the chakra imbalance may eventually lead to physical illness and other problems.

Different techniques have been developed to stimulate and balance the chakras. Some people like crystal and color therapy, others can visit a healer of energy. Meditation is, however, also a powerful and fairly easy way for chakras to be balanced, and it is particularly effective to use brainwave chakra balance meditation.

Meditation with brainwave training is a good choice, as it includes sounds of different frequencies that have been known to have a positive impact on the system of chakras and allow each chakra to vibrate to its optimum level.

Brain stimulation exercises often make it easier to reach a meditative state, as they cause brain activity to slow down when you listen-this makes them a perfect choice for someone who is not a trained meditator, and who usually has trouble relaxing and remaining calm during traditional meditation.

To use this type of stimulation chakra recording, simply sit or lie in a quiet place, focus on recording, and let it work its positive effects. Daily use of your chakra meditation is recommended because you won't automatically get perfect results right away, and in any case, most people will benefit from regular chakra tuning sessions just to keep things running smoothly.

Chakra Balancing against the Modern World

The contemporary world has brought many wonderful technological advancements but, at the same time, it has added to the lack of knowledge of the value and spiritual wellbeing of many people.

We may learn many lessons from Hindu philosophy that has held the essential role of our divine beings living in a changing environment in our overall health.

Our body contains seven centers of critical energy and several secondary centers. These power centers, known as chakras, are important for our physical, mental and spiritual health and work properly.

Our chakras have a detrimental effect on our wellbeing when they're out of control. It makes it important to preserve good health for the regeneration of the chakra. You can think of your chakras as gates that regulate the flow of energy into and out of your body. The seven major chakras draw energy from the world around you and are found in the base part of the neck from the base up to the top of your head.

What Causes the Chakras to Distort?

When your Chakras are inhibited, the flow of this energy is disrupted, and this can have a significant impact on your wellbeing, including physical health. Chakric activity can be disrupted by poor physical health and diet, stress, suppressed emotions and a variety of other factors; luckily, all of these can be reversed.

Chakra Balance is the Secret to Better Health and Satisfaction

People who have been awakened the chakras have always tried to keep them properly balanced in order to achieve high levels of physical, mental and spiritual health. Self-healing is something you might have heard of before – this is a technique that focuses on the principle of chakra balance.

Our chakras are very responsible for many aspects of our health – the functioning of our endocrine system, the diseases that may affect our health and our thinking processes. Chakra management will ensure that all functions of our physical body work properly and that our mental wellbeing is well balanced.

Chakra balancing has several advantages:

- Inner peace and a sense of well-being
- Physical health:
- Satisfactory sex life
- To be in touch with your emotions
- Increased ability to express passion
- Spiritual development and healing
- More self-confidence

There are different ways to perform chakra balancing. Try the following techniques to bring your chakras into balance:

- Therapeutic treatments-e.g. Reiki
- Yoga and meditation
- Exercise
- Light therapy
- Auric treatment of crystals and gems
- Balancing by using your hands and pendulums.
- Aromatherapy
- Therapy by touch

- Positive Thinking
- Binaural Sound Frequency
- Affirmation and Hypnosis

Our body has its own natural energy reservoir, which is used by the body and released, to be replenished by the universal energy of our chakras. The aim of chakra balancing is to ensure the efficient processing and use of this energy by the body, mind and spirit. When your chakras are restored to a healthy state, there will be inner peace and well-being. Chakra alignment takes the chakras back to a safe, balanced state.

The Importance of Balancing Your Chakras

Each of the seven (7) main chakras corresponds to the many levels of consciousness, spiritual connection, developmental stages of life, colors, sounds, and body functions of our human existence. Brainwave training is a scientifically proven technology that deliberately alters the frequency of the brain by introducing sound and/or light with a view to changing its state of consciousness. Each state of consciousness corresponds to another chakra. Practicing will activate and regulate each chakra by accessing and maintaining the frequency that resonates with that chakra.

Why It's Important to Balance Your Chakras

- When the chakra is unbalanced or out of alignment, disrupted energy can cause sickness, psychologically, physically, or emotionally.

- Blocking a chakra may result in an unexplained weakness, deficiency, or persistent discomfort in the part of the body in which it resides.

- If your heart chakra is unbalanced, you may have trouble forming close relationships, showing sympathy, or you may be too emotional to take things to heart, causing pain and worry.

- All chakras need to be open to a healthy mind, body and soul. Your well-being depends on harmony.

- If you are not balanced, feelings of peace will be foreign to you.

- Your body shape, glandular procedures, physical ailments, thoughts, and behavior can be controlled by a chakra.

- Open chakras have a good impact on all aspects of your life.

- When balanced and coordinated, you would have a greater understanding of yourself at all levels.

- Your ability to attract, assimilate and effectively direct your energy to your well-being is determined by balanced chakras.

- The more you open your chakras, the more you control your health, abundance, and happiness.

- Happy chakras allow you to feel more alive and vibrant.

- The more balanced your chakras are, the more energy you store, the more you have to use, and the more powerful you become in controlling your own individual realities.

- The less balanced your chakras, the less energy you store, resulting in a lack of inspiration, a lack of fitness, a lack of achievement, and a lack of something else of a positive nature.

The importance of balancing your chakras is essential to your overall well-being and can be easily triggered by accessing and activating each of their distinct frequencies, using brainwave training as a tool. Making sure that the "windows of your soul" are open and working, is the first step to expressing your life- force energy in the most positive way. Clearing and balancing each of your chakras will make it possible for you to live your best life.

Take advantage of the technology, brainwave training, which can easily access and sustain the frequency required to trigger the chakras. If you want to get relaxed, get focused, get energized, relax, get motivated, get clear, get connected, etc., chakra healing can be your answer to that. Your life would also feel good if your chakras are healthy. As we learn to balance our chakras, instead of living in a constant response to forces beyond ourselves, we learn to make our lives the way we want them.

These energy spirals are the healing wheels that feed the body with good energy and relieve it from what we don't want. Chakras cannot be kept, stroked or bottled like a genie, but our physical bodies are thirsty and deeply influenced by our metabolism, thoughts, perceptions and behaviors.

Furthermore to their roles in the physical realm, the chakras work on a higher plane, awakening us to the realization that our body, soul and spirit are forever and inextricably bound together.

Whether you experience stress, illness or pain, or just want to increase your energy, you're going to want to learn and practice this simple-yet-deep technique. It may be used to restore a wide variety of areas.

You just say out loud what you want to change - the problem or the pain-and stress, breathe deeply and feel the stress in

your body causing the discomfort to melt away. The idea is that you can take a deep breath and release the anxiety that disturbs your body's energy of healing by actively touching four main points of your body while reciting similar statements. It can sound basic, but the effects are also deeply life-altering.

CHAPTER FIVE

Proven Benefits Of Chakra

Chakras are strongly influenced not only by the physical and chemical factors of the environment but also by changes within the body.

They are the centers of energy, and they are the ones that give balance to our bodies. They are also vital to mental and physical activity and must, therefore, be purified. There are several ancient techniques that are used for clearing the chakra. Some of the common methods of chakra cleaning are:

- There are certain aromatic substances, such as incense sticks and herbs, which give rise to fragrance when burned. They have the ability to block harmful energies from reaching our bodies. So, this was a common process used to clean chakras.

- Auric method is another method commonly used for cleaning chakras where certain gems and crystals are used for the same purpose. The lapses of this method is that it can cause harm instead of cleaning it. Therefore, prior to carrying out this operation, it must be discussed with qualified professionals.

- If a person has a healthy diet with plenty of water, there is a possibility to clean the chakras regularly. In addition to our balanced diet, if an individual consumes fresh juice and sleeps for at least eight hours a day, the chakras would be cleaned to a greater extent.

- Regular exercise is a must for the proper functioning of the heart and cleaning of the chakras. Nature is another source to clean our chakras. So if an individual were to spend his time in the morning sunlight and the evening breeze, his chakras would be cleaned.

- Listening to music makes our mind light and refreshes our chakras.

- Meditation has the supreme power to control our senses and thus to increase the strength of our chakras. Chakra meditation is going to help you boost concentration. One great addition to meditation is the addition of binaural beats while meditating.

- In addition to all this, a person should love himself. This would give him self-confidence and incite him to live a better life.

- One should have control over one's emotions and feelings. This helps maintain our chakras and energy levels.

It may be difficult to follow all these customs. But at least one should follow what they can to keep their mind and body peaceful.

To Achieve Success

Ours is a world where people have to adapt constantly to keep up. You need to maintain a high level of motivation and energy in order to be able to do this and achieve the success that you want out of your life.

There are many ways to ensure this continuous growth in all areas – physical, mental and spiritual development are all important. Energy centers in your body play an integral part in every area of this phase of growth.

In order to succeed, you need to turn your potential energy into action; and your energy centers (or chakras) play an important role. To order to put these resources into practice, it is important that these critical energy centers are kept up to date and properly coordinated.

These chakras are located in a straight line across your body, lying along your spine. Each of these energy centers relates to a different aspect of your actions as well as to the functioning of your physical body. You should work on each energy center individually and then work to achieve the overall balance between them.

While clearing chakras, your body is capable of eliminating negative energy, taking positive energy to displace it instead.

Making movements in the counterclockwise direction helps to remove negative energy, while movement in the clockwise direction helps to generate positive energy.

There may be a little discomfort, even pain, while clearing the chakras. However, this is only energy flowing in and out, and there is nothing to be alarmed about.

These energy centers draw energy from the universe, allowing your body, mind, and spirit to energize and function more effectively.

Clearing chakras is an act that can give you new energy; some even describe it as a kind of rebirth. This cycle can be conducted as much as once a day, but it should be done at least every few weeks to maintain your chakras in peak shape.

After clearing your chakra, you will be filled with positive energy and your energy centers will be balanced. You're going to find yourself having new creative thoughts.

At first, you're going to start working on just one chakra, or maybe a few at a time. You will soon find yourself able to clear all of your chakras to achieve the potential offered by all of your untapped resources. You should have a feeling of calm and a sense of well-being.

You will know which chakras are in need of clearing and the physical manifestations that the chakras have in your body. You're going to have to learn what these are and get in tune with your chakras. When you know which parts of your physical body relate to each chakra, it will become intuitive.

Our world is competitive, and you need to be adaptable and energetic to get ahead; this means having all your energy centers in the right balance.

A growing number of people are learning that these chakras are very important to every aspect of their lives, and more and more people are working to understand how they work and to benefit.

There is a great deal of personal or individual satisfaction as well as professional achievement that can be enjoyed by those who learn how their chakras work and how to use their potential to achieve more success and a healthier life. Chakra clearing can give you the energy you need to get ahead in this ever-changing world.

Helps You Lose Weight The Sacral Chakra

Some people may experience unnatural food cravings. This, in turn, can lead to a significant increase in weight. You will need to balance your Sacred Chakra in order to deny this food craving. Here are some of the exercises that can help to keep the sacred chakra healthy.

- Dancing
- Swimming
- Indulging in good hobbies, such as healthy cooking

Ideally, to help balance your Sacred Chakra, you need to allow your body to enjoy the outer energy and imbibe it in its true flow. This will reduce the unwanted and unhealthful cravings in your body and make life easier for you.

Solar Plexus Chakra

Stress could be another major factor when it comes to weight gain. That's why you need to be sure that you're working on a chakra that can help you stay at ease and get rid of stress in your life.

The solar plexus chakra governs the ease with which you can let go of stress and stress that tends to accumulate. It's located just above the navel and below your rib cage. This chakra also helps to control blood sugar levels in the body. This is why this chakra is linked to weight loss. When you can balance the Solar Plexus Chakra, the ease with which the sugar levels are controlled in your body will increase, and that will ensure that your body stays healthy.

The Throat Chakra

The Throat Chakra is located in the area of the throat, this chakra is essentially related to communication. However, it is related to the thyroid gland and so, if the chakra is not balanced, the thyroid gland may fail to function properly and this, in turn, may lead to weight gain. So, the emphasis should be on balancing the danger chakra for smoother and more effective thyroid metabolism.

The Root Chakra

This chakra is situated and located at the base of the spine. When the Root Chakra is healthy, it will help to shed extra pounds. The weight gained in the belly area is mostly due to emotional factors. That's why it's important to balance the Root Chakra as it helps to bring emotional harmony and thus allows you to remain whole.

These are some of the ways that chakra healing can lead to weight loss and help you stay healthy. Make sure you indulge in the right forms of healing of the chakra and see how it can bring about a very positive change in your life.

INNER PACE: bridging the gap in your relationship

The heart has its reasons, reasons unknown to us. The Heart Chakra is the fourth chakra in our body, and it allows us to determine the reasons for it. Comfort in sharing emotions is something that is difficult to deny, and the success that the sharing of emotions brings is unbeatable. If you feel happy, your emotions will increase when you share that happiness with someone else. If you are unhappy, being able to share your pain, you will be comforted. If you're angry, venting your anger makes you feel better.

There was a time when we had to deal with our own conflicting emotions all by ourselves, with no one to explain, to make us understand whatever happened to us. The thought that our Heart Chakra might have been imbalanced didn't really occur to anyone. The concept of chakra healing was not common to the general public. When I was young, I was disturbed by my emotions and feelings towards a young handsome man, and I confessed to my mother about my feelings. She told me simply, "You must learn to regulate these emotions." For quite some time, I felt I was a kind of emotional freak, and I prayed that I would be flooded with better thoughts and feelings. Now, all you have to do is Google your problems, and in a matter of seconds, there are ways and means to solve them. The solution to all heart problems, one 's feelings, confusions, one's ability to feel love and hatred are all present in one center – the Heart Chakra.

The Heart Chakra affects your relationship. Its element is water, and it has the ability to relax and soothe. Like a flowing river, it calms your mind, energizes your inner self and leaves you with a calming effect like those ripples. That effect makes you want to open up to your environment, to let go of your inner pain, love, and hatred. It's what makes your heart feel like a feather. When the Heart Chakra is strong, you can enjoy a comfortable, loving and empathic relationship at home, at work and in your community. You get along with your family and the people around you who see you as a good person. You know your ethics at work; you give your best shot at all that you do. You have a deep sense of appreciation for how good your life is, and you feel compassion for those of you around you.

In fact, there is comfort in being around people who can share their emotions. Those with an open and healthy Heart Chakra let their conscious mind be aligned with their hearts to experience the feelings that give rise to a flood of feel-good hormones.

Coupling strategies and healing mechanisms, as well as techniques for balancing and achieving results, can be achieved through chakra healing. The passion that was once dead in your relationship can be resurrected in you. The flow of emotions that flow through you can be cleared up and you can feel a sense of togetherness in your relationships. Most importantly, you can feel in control of your emotions by practicing Chakra Healing and opening and empowering your Heart Chakra.

Experience the Triumph of Life

Worrying is nothing but a relentless repetition of those terms in the mind. "The inactivity of the solar plexus chakra sucks away the vitality of a person and brings the person out of the absolute consciousness and happiness of the moment.

We all face events that cause a knot in our stomach: relationships that are dysfunctional, bills that we don't have the resources to pay, job conditions that threaten our sense of strength, and sudden shifts that leave us feeling out of control of our circumstances. When our health is down and our relationships crumble, we can become so frightened that we break down.

However, if your chakras are balanced, you can feel cheerful and outgoing, and most importantly, you can have self- respect. You become more expressive and enjoy taking on new challenges with your strong sense of personal power. The body parts of this chakra include the stomach, liver, gall bladder, pancreas, and small intestines.

Chakra healing helps to open our solar plexus chakra and to strike a balance in our life. It can give us happiness and help us to fight any physical problems. The opening of the third chakra works like a miracle. It can allow you to turn a new leaf and achieve a balanced life that everyone wants.

Soothing the Migraines

One of the chakras is located in the head, specifically in the center of the forehead, between the eyes, called the Brow Chakra. This is also known as the Third Eye. In Sanskrit, this chakra is known as the Anja and is the sixth of the seven primary chakras. This chakra is said to be connected to the psychic abilities. Physically, it is linked to the pineal and pituitary glands.

The other chakra in the head is called the Sahasrara or the Thousand-Petaled Lotus. This is more widely known as the Crown Chakra since it is situated on the top of the head and covers the entire crown area. The function of this chakra is to regulate the flow of energy through the body. If this chakra is blocked or experienced imbalance, tension, sleep issues, exhaustion and migraine are said to occur.

Many of the techniques used to align the chakras include meditation, visualization and color therapy. But there is no assurance that the migraines will leave permanently. That's why it's vital to find a real basis for the problem and attack it with a genuine natural solution that will stop your migraine headaches [http:/stop-a-migraine-headache.com].

Energizing Yourself by Chakra Meditation

Inside our bodies, there are points of energy that we use that will allow us to fully experience and realize the world around us. These are usually points of light that are made up of rainbow colors. They are called chakras.

Each color chakra reflects and is found in various areas of the body, such as the head and the stomach. Many organs within the chakra region are specifically influenced by the properties of the chakra.

Although each chakra has a purpose, it also needs to be strengthened. That's where meditation is the key. You will find various websites and books not only talking about the chakras and their purposes but also how to exercise them so that they can work for you.

Usually, the method of meditation involves sitting or lying down, taking a deep breath and focusing on each chakra in your body. As you do, you imagine that the color of that chakra is emitted as a ray of light and often followed by a symbol to help you focus more on this chakra.

For example, the Sacral Chakra, which is located in the lower abdomen, is represented by the color orange. So, if you prefer, you can imagine an orange beam coming out of your body or through your body. Instead, you can imagine a symbol or representation of that chakra. Because it is represented by joy and giving and receiving, you can imagine that you have received a lovely orange fabric.

So, while you may not have been able to think about the image or representation of the Sacral Chakra or the orange color associated with it, you might want to see the crystals and gems of amber or coral that are said to represent it. In addition to imagining the colors of each chakra that you shoot out of your body, you might also want to imagine that your body and mind are cleansing themselves from the clutter or issues that might affect your chakras.

For example, the Heart Chakra, located in the center of the chest, is symbolized by love and understanding, as well as forgiveness, balance and compassion. If you have been feeling out of balance or someone has recently hurt you and you feel bad feelings or pain in this area, it is more than likely that this chakra is blocked and a chakra-related issue needs to be examined or looked at.

While you become more aware of the chakras in your meditation practice, you can also become more aware of the issues involved and find clarity on how to better deal with these issues. Not only will you clear yourself, but your body, mind, and spirit will thank you for that.

Helps Remove Negative Thoughts

Negative thoughts, from old childhood programming, which are held in the subconscious mind, can be removed and overridden by the creation of new positive neural networks of thought.

The chakras are the portal to your mind. Having access to your chakras can tell you a lot about what's going on in your life and how you're living it.

Chakras are involved in all your physical, mental, emotional and spiritual processes.

If any of these chakras become unbalanced or out of tune, the lack of energy flow can cause disease at any or all of these levels. If your chakras are not balanced, you will have no lasting sense of peace. The imbalance in the movement of energy through the chakra results in an imbalance in the overall healthy functioning of the body.

Chakras are having an effect on your life. When the chakra spins smoothly, you're in good alignment. You're blocked when it's obstructed.

How Negative Thinking Blocks a Chakra

There's a reaction to every thought. Whether it energizes you or reduces your life-force depends on your thinking. If you think there's a negative thought, it changes the electricity in the brain, which changes the message. Due to changes in the brain, the energy at the meridians (the spine and through your head, where the energy is running through) is changing.

The organs connected to the meridian do not obtain the vital energy they need, and the disease develops. Universal energy input changes in the chakra due to negative thought and takes you out of touch with the universe, and a barrier happens.

Negative thinking takes energy away from your subtle auric body. If you are at alert, you can see that the colors are dim. Your auric shield is weakening, and outside negative energy can be poured into you.

When you send negative thoughts to the environment, that's what you're going to attract, but it's even stronger. Increasing chakra is associated with a specific part of the body, and when balanced, allowing energy to flow freely gives you a sense of well-being. If the body has a sense of well-being, the mind should have a sense of well-being.

Brainwave training is one of many ways to develop your chakras so that they can hold and disperse energy freely, remove any negative thoughts that may block them, and replace them with positive thoughts. Clearing and balancing each of your chakras will make it possible for you to live your best life.

Helps balance your prosperity

Entrainment re-programs your brain with constructive thought processes that restore the cellular brain of your initial success consciousness that you were born with. This scientifically proven technological tool uses sound to influence the main frequency of brain waves, and gives you back your God-given ability to manifest prosperity and abundance, health and happiness.

A blocked prosperity chakra does not normally occur in response to a single event, but rather a series of similar events over time, without relief. The health of this chakra depends on whether you have received unconditional love and affection for the first three years of your life. If you haven't, chances are that your prosperity or root chakra will be blocked, and abundance and prosperity is not something you're used to.

Sign Your Prosperity Chakra Is Unbalanced or Blocked

- You talk about pessimistic feelings.
- You're always scared of most things.
- There are problems with constipation, hemorrhoids, the intestine, the large intestine, and the digestive system.
- You have problems with your lower back, the base of your spine, legs and feet, bone and/or dental disorders, poor overall health and lack of vitality and energy.
- You may be obese
- You have osteoarthritis.
- You have severe mood swings.
- You're having trouble living right now.
- You are disconnected and alienated from others.
- You can't manifest—any good thing.
- You can encounter autoimmune diseases such as lupus, arthritis, multiple sclerosis, thyroid disorders, AIDS, cancer, and allergies — when the body attacks itself.
- You have depression that suppresses the immune system.

- You have problems with fertility.

- You have issues of prosperity.

- If you are a woman, you can't have an orgasm, and if you are a male, you will suffer from premature ejaculation.

- You have leg and foot cramps.

- If possible, you cannot let go of your sorrow or material sources of comfort.

- You are unable to release or move forward.

If this chakra is blocked or unbalanced, there is a power disturbance that can be re-opened and balanced if you have access to the right frequency. Brainwave training will reach the frequency and is a simple and quick way to begin the healing process of the happiness chakra and all the other chakras above it.

This chakra is the foundation of your life, and the health of all the other chakras depends on their balance. Clearing and balancing each of your chakras will make it possible for you to live your best life. Take advantage of the technology, brainwave training, that can easily access and maintain the frequency needed to activate the chakras.

Gemstone Therapy and Central Chakra Channel

Gemstone Therapy can be a key to enlivening the central chakra channel. The central chakra channel is a stream of energy that runs along the spine and is meant to feed the chakras. The main chakra channel in the Eastern Teachings is called the shushumna nadi. Ideally, it's about three to five inches wide. It extends from the Earth Star Chakra (the 11th Chakra, located in the ground below our feet), through the 7th chakras, all the way through the 8th, 9th, and 10th chakras, far above the top of the head.

One aim of this channel is to unite the energies of the earth and the heavens, which will become a source of nourishment for all chakras. The energy of the planet travels up the channel from the bottom of the channel, and the energy of the heavens joins it from the top. Within it, the energy mixes to the exact proportions that each chakra needs. Healthy chakras have roots that reach this channel from the vortex of the chakra to receive this nourishment.

Many individual central chakra channels are in very poor health. Let's examine some common anomalies that can occur. The channel can be withered to as much as half an inch in diameter. It may have blockages or constrictions over certain chakras. The energy moving through the channel can be slow, ineffective, and, in some cases, non-existent. Roots of the chakra may be absent or withered and thin and receive only minimal nourishment. The structure of the canal may be intact, but there may be no movement of earth and the energy of heaven flowing through it.

Ideally, the central chakra channel should provide a warm spring of nourishment that is so refreshing and enticing that every chakra will build and maintain its roots in order to access this channel and its vitalizing content. In short, the chakras can be as good as the central channel that feeds them.

Gemstone Energy Medicine provides a way to rebuild, create and preserve your core channel. The tanzanite gemstone has a natural affinity to this channel. Its heating energy relaxes the tension in the channel and invites it to open up. White beryllium, in combination with tanzanite, clears and purifies the channel. When the blue sapphire is added to these gemstones, the vibrations of the channel are lifted and become more receptive to the earth and the energies of heaven.

If you wear these gemstones in a therapeutic gemstone necklace, the irregularities of the chakras are fixed naturally and gently over time. However, energy workers can use this combination in certain gemstone therapy techniques to treat different types of central channel anomalies directly during a gemstone therapy session.

Enhanced Communication

Communication is not limited to the sharing of conversation between two people but is far more than that. There are many forms of communication, including your gestures, body language, symbols and sign language, etc. Communication can be multidimensional using facial expressions or silence to convey messages. There is another aspect of the throat chakra called the inner voice. Our inner voice is a channel of our own emotions, feelings, perceptions, knowledge, and higher spiritual powers. The associated sound is "HAM" and if you chant this regularly, you can open the chakra or clear any blockage. There are other techniques, such as color therapy, that help to open the chakra. The color associated with this chakra is blue. If one of your chakras doesn't work properly, you feel weak and distorted.

For many years, a lot of people have been focusing on meditation as a method of opening up all of our body's chakras, and it has proved to be silently effective. Concentrate with your eyes closed on the chakra that you feel is blocked and purify with the energy generated within your body.

Our energy bodies are helping us to feel and express ourselves. View more about the chakras gives us a better understanding of ourselves. It is very important to open the throat chakra to convey and interact with others in a more free and clear manner. Awareness brings us closer to ourselves and gives us the power to heal ourselves and others.

When our chakras are well balanced and clear, it affects our emotional, spiritual and physical well-being. Chakra clearing is a wonderful tool for a healthy lifestyle. When an imbalance occurs in any of the seven different parts, the overall sense of the inner self is ruined. Increasing chakra is linked to a variety of problems and a range of meditation techniques offer solutions to solve them.

Muladhara: Red/ Earth:

This part of the chakra is centered around the spinal base. It is known to be the most important chakra. Well, it can be related to one's survival instincts and one's physical identity. You can use this chakra to make you healthy and safe.

Svadhisthan: Orange/Water

This is the center of emotional and sexual desires. This chakra is found in the lower back and in the abdomen and brings us closer to each other. Focusing on this chakra will improve your emotional control, sexual satisfaction and your ability to change.

Anahata: Green/Air

Anahata brings inner peace and love to you. It concerns the heart and opposites, such as the male and the female, and the mind and the body. It brings you to a state of self-acceptance, too.

Manipur: Yellow /Fire

This chakra is about your ego identity. It also corresponds to the power of your will. It is responsible for the metabolism of the body. You're going to get strength and energy by meditating on this chakra.

Vishuddha: Blue/Sound:

The chakra is the core of creativity. It allows you to express yourself. As it is located in the throat, it represents vibrations, tongues and sounds.

Ajna: Light/Purple

Ajna allows people to think and see more clearly. It's also known as the third eye. It stands for light and reflection. It helps you to see better both physically and mentally.

Sahasrara: Violet/Pension

While this is not considered superior to other chakras, it is the only chakra with a profound relation to the universe beyond.

This chakra gives you the happiness, the spirituality, the wisdom of the unknown. It's linked to thought and self- consciousness. It's called the crown of the body.

The trick to practicing chakra meditation is to understand all the chakras and what they say. If all your chakras are aligned, you will hit the Sahasrara level, which will give you a deeper understanding of life. This is going to bring you peace and happiness. After studying all seven parts of this exercise, you will seek to establish mastery of each of them.

Conclusion

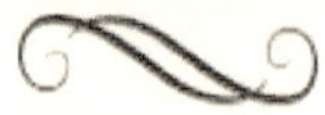

In concluding this book, let's briefly examine the seven main chakras in our energy system. This is a brief summary of what we've learned, and we can use it as a checklist to see how we may do it. The chakras are a vast study, and we've only looked briefly, but that's enough for us to get to work on each chakra and improve all aspects of our lives.

The chakras are circular vortexes or energy wheels, depicted as flowers with petals spinning and vibrating. There are several chakras, but we looked at the key seven for energy healing research. They start with the first chakra on our tail bone and finish with the seventh at the crown of our head. They are the focal points of our life force or energy, and the state of each chakra is vital to our overall health and well- being.

If we face many challenges in a particular area of our life, then it is most likely that the chakra concerned with this part of our life is dysfunctional, may even be closed. So, it is up to us to open up and strengthen the chakra so that we can heal the situation. We are energy beings with unlimited potential, so we just need to educate ourselves and use our own power and knowledge to create what we want or want in our lives.

Today, we're increasingly conscious of healing our lives with natural systems and chakra healing's ancient science holds the secret to almost everything in life that we might ever want.

Thank you, I hope you enjoyed the book.

Crystals For Beginners

The Complete Guide To Understand And Practice The Healing Power Of Crystals

CARLISLE PALMER

Introduction

A crystal is a material whose constituents (such as atoms, molecules, or ions) are arranged in a microscopic structure that is high in its order, forming a crystal lattice that extends in all paths. It is also called a crystalline solid. Besides this, single macroscopic crystals are usually identifiable by their geometric shape, consisting of flat faces with specific orientations of character. The scientific study of crystals and the formation of crystals is called crystallography. The crystal formation process via crystal growth mechanisms is called the crystallization or solidification process.

The word crystal is from the ancient Greek word (krustallos), meaning "ice" as well as "rock crystal," "icy cold, frost." Popular crystal samples include diamonds, snowflakes, and table salt. Most crystals are inorganic solids, but polycrystals are several microscopic crystals fused into one solid together. Many of these like ceramics, minerals, and ice are good examples of polycrystals. The third category of solids is amorphous solids, where the atoms have no periodic structure. Amorphous solids such as wax, glass, and many plastics are examples.

Notwithstanding the term, lead crystal, crystal glass, and related products are not crystals but rather glass forms, i.e., amorphous solids. Crystals are often used in pseudoscientific practices such as crystal therapy, and in Wiccan beliefs and related religious movements, along with gemstones, and are sometimes associated with spell work.

The scientific definition of a "crystal" is based on the microscopic arrangement of the atoms within it, called the structure of crystals. A crystal is stable, in which the atoms form a regular agreement. Not all the crystals are solids. For example, when liquid water begins to freeze, the change in phase begins with small ice crystals forming until they fuse, forming a polycrystalline structure. Each of the tiny crystals (called "crystallites or grains") in the final form of ice is a pure gem with a periodic arrangement of atoms. The entire polycrystal does not have a natural method since the regular pattern at the grain boundaries is broken. Many inorganic macroscopic solids are polycrystalline, like almost all the metals, ice, ceramics, rocks, etc. Solids that are neither crystalline nor polycrystalline, such as glass, are referred to as amorphous solids.

These may not have a periodic, even microscopic order. There are significant distinctions between crystalline solids and amorphous solids: the process of forming a glass most noticeably does not release the latent heat of fusion but instead constitutes a crystal. A crystal structure is (an arrangement of atoms in a crystal) distinguished by its unit cell, a small imaginary box in a specific spatial arrangement that contains one or more atoms. To get the gem, the unit cells are stack in tri-dimensional space.

The requirement limit in a crystal's symmetry is that the unit cells stack perfectly, without any gaps. There are 219 possible symmetries of crystals, called crystallographic groupings of space. Crystal systems have seven groups, the cubic crystal system where crystals can form rectangular boxes or cubes, such as Halite (mineral) or the hexagonal crystal system (where crystals can form hexagons, such as ordinary water ice).

There are several ways to use crystals to help heal, enrich, and sustain you through the journey of life. Our in-depth articles explore several of such ways to tap into these energies and how to preserve and care for more sensitive crystals in your collected works. You will learn how you can use the crystal energies to support your physical bodies and understand how these stones have a close link to your chakras and higher self in general.

We will discuss not only how each type of crystal is unique, but also how every single piece of the same kind of crystal is distinctive in itself. You can learn how to tap into these healing energies and calming powers, and how to use crystals to activate your latent energies and spiritual prowess. Through us, you'll also discover how specific colors evoke certain emotions and meanings. Purple crystals tend to be highly psychic and spiritual. Red stones often have to do with our passions, our circulation, hearts, and health, and blue rocks often promote clarity of mind, clear communication, etc.

Each stone has its energies and strengths, but don't feel overwhelmed just yet. You will find your intuition to be a helpful guide, and of course, you will feel excited and curious about some of the stones that we are discussing that you know will work best for you.

CHAPTER ONE

Crystal Faces And Shapes

Crystals are widely recognized by their shape, which consists of flat, sharp, angled faces. For a gem, these shape features are not necessary — a crystal is scientifically defined by its atomic microstructural arrangement, not its macroscopic shape — but the characteristic macroscopic shape is often present and easy to see.

Euhedral crystals are those with visible flat faces that are well-shaped. Anhedral crystals are not, typically, because the gem in a polycrystalline solid is one grain.

A euhedral crystal's flat faces (also called facets) are in a particular way relative to the crystal's underlying atomic arrangement: planes with relatively low Miller index. It happens because some surface orientations are more stable than others (less energy from the surface). As a crystal grows, new atoms easily attach themselves to the surface's rougher and less durable parts but less easily to the flat, secure surfaces. Therefore, the flat surfaces tend to grow bigger and smoother until these plane surfaces consist of the entire crystal surface. One of the oldest techniques in crystallography research is to calculate the three-dimensional orientations of a crystal's faces and use them to infer the underlying symmetry of crystals. The habit of a crystal is its outer visible form. It is the crystal structure (which limits potential facet orientations), the particular crystal chemistry and bonding (which may benefit certain facets over others), and the situations under which the crystal is created.

Occurrence in Nature

Rocks

The highest concentrations of crystals on Earth are part of its solid bedrock by volume and weight. Typically, crystals found in rocks range in size from a fraction of a millimetre to several centimetres across, although huge crystals sometimes found. A gem of beryl from Madagascar, Malakialina, 18 m (59 ft) long and 3.5 m (11 ft) in diameter, weighing 380,000 kg (840,000 lb), was the largest known naturally occurring crystal in the world as of 1999.

The vast majority of igneous rocks is formed from molten magma, and the degree of crystallization primarily depends on the conditions in which they solidified. An example of the stones is granite, which crystallizes completely and cools very gradually and under high pressure. Other kinds of lava are poured out at the surface and cooled very quickly, and a small amount of glassy or amorphous matter is typical in this latter category. Other crystalline rocks are recrystallizing, the metamorphic rocks such as marbles, mica-schists, and quartzites. It indicates that they were at first fragmentary rocks like calcareous, shale, and sandstone and were never in molten form or entirely in solution.

Other rock crystals form druses or quartz veins out of precipitation from fluids, usually water. Evaporites such as gypsum, Halite (mineral), and some calcareous stones were deposited from aqueous solution, mainly due to arid climate evaporation.

Ice

Snow, sea ice, and glaciers dependent on the water are growing crystalline/polycrystalline systems on Earth and other planets. A single snowflake is an individual or a series of crystals, whereas a polycrystal is an ice cube.

Organigenic Crystals

Many living organisms can produce crystals, such as calcite and aragonite or hydroxylapatite, in most molluscs or vertebrates.

Crystal Growth

Crystal growth is when a pre-existing crystal becomes larger due to more growth units (e.g., molecules, ions) being added in their crystal lattice positions, or a solution developed into a gem or further growth being processed. A crystal is defined as atoms, molecules, or ions arranged in an orderly pattern of repetition, a crystal lattice extending into all three dimensions of space. Thus, crystal growth differs from the growth of a liquid droplet in that the ions or molecules must fall into the correct lattice positions during growth to grow a well-ordered crystal. The diagram provides a basic example of a gem increasing with a simple cubic lattice, by adding a molecule.

When, in a perfect crystal lattice, the molecules or ions fall into positions different from those, crystal defects form. Usually, in a crystal lattice, the molecules or ions are stuck in the sense that they cannot move from their locations. Thus, crystal growth is always permanent once the ions or molecules have fallen into place in the expanding lattice.

Mechanisms of growth

At temperatures below the melting point, the interface between a crystal and its vapor can be molecularly sharp. An ideal crystalline surface grows by spreading single layers, or equivalently by advancing laterally in the growth steps that connected the layers. This technique uses a finite driving force (or degree of supercooling) to lower the nucleation barrier sufficiently for nucleation to occur through thermal fluctuations in perceptible growth rates. Burton and Cabrera have distinguished between two essential mechanisms in the theory of crystal growth from the molt.

Non-uniform lateral growth

The surface progresses by the lateral movement of steps, which are one interplanar height spacing (or some integral multiple of it). A surface entity undergoes no shift and does not generally progress to itself except during the passing of a step, and then it advances by the height of a level. It is useful to understand the phase as a transformation of a surface between two adjacent regions parallel to each other and thus identical in configuration — replaced by an integral number of lattice planes. Note the distinct possibility of a phase in a diffuse surface here, although the step height will be much smaller than the thin surface thickness.

Uniform normal growth

The surface usually progresses by itself, without the need for a mechanism of gradual development. It means that each cover is capable of continuous change, contributing to the advancement of the interface in the presence of an adequate thermodynamic driving force; For a discontinuous or sharp surface, each new layer can make these changes more or less uniform over large areas. For a more diffuse cover, a mechanism of continuous growth may require simultaneous modification over several successive layers.

Non-uniform lateral growth is a geometric phase movement — as opposed to the progress of the entire surface, which is natural to itself. Alternatively, average uniform growth is based on the time sequence of a surface element. There is no motion or transition in this mode, even if a move is made through a continuous change. To understand crystal growth, the prediction of which its mechanism will be operational under any given set of conditions, is essential. For this predict, two criteria are used:

- If the surface is diffused or not: a diffuse cover is one where the transition from one phase to another is constant, occurring on many atomic planes. It contrasts to a sharp edge for which the significant property change (e.g., density or composition) is discontinuous and is usually confined to a depth of one interplanar distance.

- Whether the surface is unique or not: a singular surface is one in which the surface tension has a pointed minimum as a function of orientation. Extraordinary surface growth is known to require steps, whereas non-singular covers are generally considered to be able to progress typically to themselves.

Driving force

Consider next the required lateral growth appearance criteria. The lateral growth mechanism can be found when any area on the surface in the presence of a driving force can reach a metastable equilibrium. It will then continue to stay in such a configuration of balance until one phase passes. The design will be the same afterward except that each part of the step itself will have advanced by the height of the stage. If the surface cannot achieve equilibrium in the presence of a driving force, it will continue to proceed without the lateral movement of measures.

Thus, Cahn concluded that the distinctive feature is the surface's ability to reach a state of equilibrium in the presence of the driving force. He also found that there is a critical driving force for any exterior or interface in a crystalline medium, which, if exceeded, will allow the surface or interface to progress normally to itself, and will require the lateral growth mechanism if not exceeded.

Thus, the interface can move uniformly for sufficiently large driving forces without either heterogeneous nucleation or screw dislocation mechanism being beneficial. What constitutes a large enough driving force depends on the interface's diffuseness so that this critical driving force will be so small for extremely diffuse interfaces that any measurable driving force will exceed that. Alternatively, the essential driving force for sharp interfaces will be very high, and the lateral phase mechanism will generate the most development.

The thermo-dynamic driving force is determined by the degree of super-cooling in a crystallization phase.

Crystal Morphology

Mechanical and other properties of crystals are also generally believed to be relevant to the subject matter, and crystal morphology provides the missing link between growth kinetics and physical properties. The necessary thermodynamic device offers the study of heterogeneous equilibrium by Josiah Willard Gibbs. He provided a specific description of surface energy, making the principle of surface tension applicable to both solids and liquids. He also appreciated that a non-spherical equilibrium shape implied by anisotropic surface free energy be described thermodynamically as the form minimizes total surface free energy.

It may be instructive to note that whisker growth provides the connection between the high strength mechanical phenomenon in whiskers and the various mechanisms of growth that are responsible for their fibrous morphologies. (The single-crystal whiskers had the highest tensile strength of any known materials prior to the discovery of carbon nanotubes). Many processes produce defect-free whiskers while others may have single-screw dislocations along the main growth axis — creating whiskers with high power.

The mechanism behind growth of whiskers is not well known, but compressive mechanical stresses, including mechanically induced stresses, stresses prompted by diffusion of different materials, and thermally induced stresses, tend to be encouraged. In some ways, metal whiskers vary from metal dendrites. Dendrites are as fern-shaped as a tree's leaves, and expand over the metal surface. Whiskers, by comparison, are fibrous and extend at the right angle to the growth surface, or substratum.

Diffusion-control

Very often when the super-saturation (or degree of super-cooling) is high, and often even when not high, the kinetics of growth can be regulated by diffusion. The polyhedral crystal form will be unstable under such conditions, it will sprout protrusions at its edges and corners where the degree of supersaturation is at its highest level. The tips of such protrusions are simply the highest level of supersaturation. It is commonly assumed that the protrusion should get longer (and thinner at the tip) until the effect of free interfacial energy in growing the chemical potential reduces the growth of the tip and retains a constant value for the thickness of the tip.

A corresponding instability of the shape should occur in the subsequent tip-thickening process. It will exaggerate small bumps or bulges and expand into increasingly growing side branches. A minor degree in anisotropy should be sufficient in such an unstable or meta-stable situation to determine directions of significant branching and growth. Of course, this claim's most appealing feature is that it yields the primary morphological characteristics of dendritic development.

Choosing Your Crystal Shape

You might wonder if your crystal's shape matters. Although your crystal's healing properties should stay the same regardless of form, the experience you have with your crystal will vary. Then you'll find some of the most common crystal forms, and how to work with them:

Element

A crystal point is an excellent tool of energy that focuses and amplifies the stone's power. You can use it to channel inward healing energy, by turning the point toward you, or by turning it away from you. Many people use their positions to manifest wishes, and even after you leave the world, a standing point will continue to radiate the strength of your purpose. Due to their flexibility, points are some of the best crystals for beginners.

Sphere

A sphere of crystals emits energy in every direction in equal measure. It provides gentle, full power in which you can feel both grounded and plunged. In meditation, holding two spheres brings a sense of harmony to your practice.

Cube

Related to the root chakra is a crystal cube. It makes the creation of calmness in your environment a powerfully grounding stone. You can set up a defensive grid by putting a crystal cube in each of your room's four corners — do not worry, we'll go deeper through what grids are in a little bit.

Pyramid

Pyramids are a pure form used in many ancient civilizations. Use a crystal pyramid to beam energy concentrated up into the universe. Use it to help manifest your thoughts by writing them down on paper and placing the pyramid of crystal on top.

Heart

This loving crystal shape is great to remind you to keep it close at heart for its healing properties. Work with them to fill your soul with the energy you wish to give and receive.

Harmonizers

Crystal harmonizers are a pair of cylinder-shaped crystals that help you put your meditation into spiritual, mental, and physical balance.

Cluster

Crystal clusters are one of nature's most important occurrences. When a lot of points form on the same matrix, a cluster happens. Because there are so many points on a cluster, higher energy is believed to vibrate; having a cluster in your home will ensure it stays uplifted with the energy you want to expand.

Tumbled Stones

Tumbled stones are celebrated for their vast array of uses. They can easily hold in your pocket or purse, as small, smooth rocks. You can use these to build your crystal grids as well. Tumbled stones are one of the best crystals for beginners if you're new to this, and you're trying to decide which crystals work best for you.

What's a Crystal Grid?

Sometimes we get so caught explaining why some stones or crystal shapes are ideal for crystal grids, that we don't all know what a grid is! But let's downplay it. A crystal grid is a type of stone that usually emanates from one central stone. Grids are useful for intentionally creating energy, and holding that energy long after you set it. These arrangements of crystal grids fuse the powers of several crystals into a symphony of harmonizing vibrations. Grids can be small, take up just a tiny portion of your desk or sacred altar, or they might be massive, like the crystal grid we decided to visit on our spiritual retreat in Kauai that was big enough for us to lay down in the center.

How to Create Your Crystal Grid?

Using your intuition to create your crystal grid is the best way. Comprehend what energy you want to develop and work from there. Although there is no correct way to build a network, we prefer to use a crystal point in our middle as it helps to combine the many energies of the stones and intensify the unified energy into space. Also, if you use a grid fabric, you can find it easier to map your grid, so you are assured of the symmetry.

Pick those that align with your purpose when selecting your stones. So, you should select stones like jade, pyrite, aventurine, goldstone, citrine, and tiger's eye for a crystal grid for money. At the same time, you would choose the stones rose quartz, rhodochrosite, malachite, carnelian, rhodonite, amazonite, and jasper Kambala for a crystal grid for love. You would want their energy-filtered after you have your crystals. Clean both your crystals and space with sages or palo santo smoke. Then write on a piece of paper your intention, fold it, say the intention aloud, and put the material under the center stone. Then fill in the residual grid. Activate the crystal by taking a quartz point and draw an invisible line connecting each stone in the grid while you imagine your plan's fruitfulness.

How to Cleanse Your Crystals?

We cannot talk to beginners about the basics of crystals, without emphasizing the importance of crystal cleansing. If you never cleanse your crystals, their energy will eventually become overloaded and dim. Here are some natural methods for cleaning the crystals:

- Sage or Palo Santo Smoke — Immerse it in the smoke of a sage or palo santo to purify the crystal's energy. Perform regular crystal cleaning, or whenever your crystal begins to feel like it doesn't vibrate with the same energy it once did.

- Sun or Moon Light — Crystal cleansing can also be done by leaving your crystal out in the sun or moonlight for at least 4 hours.

- Earth's soil — Burrow your stones in the earth's land or even the potted plant's earth for up to 24 hours. Don't forget to leave a marker to remember where you put it!

- Quartz or Selenite Crystal — Quartz and selenite are two of the best beginner crystals because they are both crystals that clean. Cleaning crystals are high-vibration purifiers that need not be charged. You can use them to load and clean your other crystals because their energy remains clear and amplified. Place a stone on your cleansing crystal to purify its energy and improve it.

CHAPTER TWO

Types Of Crystal

Abalone Shell

Abalone Shell is a protective stone with a beautiful ocean-like color, not least because it serves this same literal function in nature. At times when you seem to lose your faith, or you feel insecure, find your Abalone Shell for guidance and warmth.

This stone is a trendy one in overcoming anxiety and in remaining true to oneself, particularly in heart matters. If you often feel that your relationships get in the way of fear and self-sabotage, this might be the stone for you.

Agate Crystal

Agate works because it connects to you for a broader viewpoint, and it lets you see all pros and cons of every situation. This makes it an excellent stone for us who are looking to enter a new chapter of life – a new relationship, a new career move, and so on – with confidence and security.

Agate has been heralded as a stone of considerable balance and grounding energy for centuries. There is a great sense of positivity inside Agate, indicating that even the most pessimistic and exhausted people in the world among us can find some hope for the future by letting in the energies of this stone.

Amazonite.

There is an abundant amount of love and healing energy in Amazonite that can help break cycles of negative thoughts that you may encounter throughout your life. Amazonite can also aid in unusually notable cases to reveal things, and breakthrough karmic habits left over from lifetimes and prior incarnations.

Amazonite usually is seen as a stone of bravery – perhaps apt when one considers warriors of the Amazons! It will awaken you to your courage and help you stand firmly but compassionately when you break the illusions that keep you going through the same mistakes repeatedly.

Amethyst

Ever a guiding light for psychic practitioners, and also a beautiful crystal for use in jewelry, Amethyst is popular as well as influential. It can awaken you to higher knowledge and bind you to guidance from outside the physical world, but for physical healing, it is just as powerful as a stone. Amethyst also has an aura of tranquillity about it, as well as an energy for soothing headaches and joint pain. Because of this, it is good crystal for stress relief, and to stop your mind from cycling again and again through the same handful of worries, disrupting sleep and concentration.

Apatite

Ambition and a feeling of enthusiasm for life are all amplified when the Apatite energies come into your life. This stone has a beautiful color, which also improves clarity in your mind, and it can be interesting to sit with a piece and look at the patterns created in its natural makeup.

Apatite is seen as an excellent stone for creative thinking, meaning it's okay not only for those who work in the media and the arts but also for scientists and business people to unlock new out of the box thinking. This is a versatile stone, with plenty for all areas of life to offer.

Apophyllite

Apophyllite is an excellent stone for calming an overactive mind, with its frosty white and cool blue hues. It can also help prevent any bad behaviors, such as nervous twitches and tics, that are overly energized.

But apophyllite is a stone about prevention as much as it is a cure. It functions by bringing to light the root causes of certain behaviors and sparse patterns of life. It is not always an easy process, but spiritual growth and soul development must enter new phases. Also, this stone helps relieve the strain of specific changes.

Aquamarine

Aquamarine, as the name suggests, is a stone highly connected to water and its healing, nutritious properties. In this stone, you may feel as if the essence of life awaits you, so often, its healing energies can be intense.

But this is also a stone about the tides of life-change. When you have difficulty moving on from stressful circumstances and relationships, Aquamarine ties you to your inner power. It can also help you align with others who are on the same journey.

Aragonite

Aragonite is a great gem to have if you wish to forge a deeper Earth connection. Aragonite is a crystal that will make you feel profoundly embedded in our world, releasing excess energy, centering yourself, and silencing your mind.

During times of stress, its grounding and stabilizing energies would be beneficial. It will keep you from making wild emotion-based decisions. And it will foster focus and enhance concentration.

Aventurine

Aventurine is a crystal that is connected firmly to the chakra of the heart, and that is where a lot of old sayings are born about following one's heart. Yet these energies, in keeping with the adventurous sounding nature of the name of this crystal, inspire you to be daring enough to follow your heart.

There's a sense of taking a playful risk with Aventurine. Many have called it the Stone of the Gambler, claiming it binds you with good fortune and lucky streaks. Belief in luck differs from one to another; it hardly hurts to have a little extra good luck coming one's way!

Azurite

Azurite is also referred to as the Stone of the Heavens, making it a common choice for those who strive to follow divine guidance and connections to the angelic realm. This is a crystal that helps open one's mind to what a strictly pragmatic mentality would find impossible.

It is a stone of faith and belief in something outside of oneself. However, with just as much power, it also promotes confidence in oneself, and it can help you through on vibrant ideas as and when they strike, confident of your success. Even this stone is good to clear off tension and worry.

Black Tourmaline

Like other crystals that share its color and density, Black Tourmaline is something of a guardian stone that protects you from harmful energies. Therefore, the crystal has become especially popular with natural empaths or people otherwise inclined to pick up on other's emotions and energies. Black Tourmaline is a mighty barrier between you and others, making sure you can't get dragged into drama or emotional blackmail. It is the right booster of confidence! The more you learn to work with its energies, the Black Tourmaline can also protect places and others.

Bloodstone

Bloodstone is very much on your side, despite its perhaps provocative name, as you will discover if you are working with it for crystal healing. It can help alleviate all sorts of physical pain and injuries, as well as boost the adequate circulation of both the bloodstream and the energy centers of your spirit body.

Bloodstone is connected to the base chakra, which in physical reality, is what anchors you most. It is a stone in which to enjoy the moment, then, and experience the pleasures of life. However, it is also a powerful anchoring stone when used in meditation that stops you from wandering too far into the ethereal realm.

Blue Lace Agate Stone

It is a soothing and friendly stone, even though one thinks only of its colors. Blue Lace Agate has a magical look, and the way light plays off even the most straightforward piece of it has a lot of meaning. This crystal is related to your ability to articulate and form your ideas. This crystal will help you if you still find that you are punishing yourself for not standing up against unjust practices, or turning down favors asked of you when you know they are too overreaching. It will inspire firm and not compassionate words that convey your point and help you see that most people who make such requests are not trying to be unkind to you.

Bronzite

While many crystals are specialized, to one or the other chakras of your inner energy, bronzite is one of those comparatively harder to find gems that speak to all your chakras. It aligns them and helps you figure out which facets of yourself that need healing and focus.

Bronzite, however, is a stone that has a lot of defensive qualities too. It helps you know when people want to pull the wool over your head, but it can also help activate your immune system's more reliable parts. The dreaded office disease that seems to spread all of a sudden will affect you much less often!

Carnelian

Carnelian's vibrant orange might look like sunset warmth, but this is one stone that will consider leaving you anything but tired. This stone has a powerful undercurrent of vitality that benefits and electrifies your thoughts with ideas and ambitions.

Carnelian is also attached to your sacral chakra, where you feel and process many of the pleasures of life. If you have experienced a little less passion for life than usual, Carnelian is just the stone you need to reinvigorate that joie de vivre, and to succeed you have to chomp at the bit.

Chrysocolla Colla

As far as transformation goes in life, it is generally either our desire or that life-forcing events shift over us – often with or without our permission! And in the case of Chrysocolla, with divine encouragement, you can find that you will encourage a positive shift in your life.

This crystal and the colors of its rich earth also marvellously bind you to the natural world. Just as the seasons roll in cycles, you will also see the cycles for what they are in your own life and feel empowered to nurture or break those cycles following your needs.

Chrysoprase

Though it may seem a pure pale green stone at first appearance, Chrysoprase has many hidden depths. It could be that this is one crystal, which is also ideal for getting to the bottom of some of yours.

It is a stone of truth and enlightenment, meaning you will see behind other people's lies and stop kidding yourself in some areas of life. Thanks to the strong concepts of redemption and love flowing through the energies of this stone, it's excellent for healing and solving problems.

Citrine

Vibrant in color, as well as in its energies, Citrine is a crystal that cannot help but encourage positivity and resolve. It interacts with your solar plexus chakra, where most people share enthusiasm, as well as some intuitive wisdom – or 'positive feelings,' as we sometimes call them.

But Citrine also promotes the idea of growth alongside strengthening those parts of ourselves. Be it an individual's growth, a relationship's growth, financial prosperity growth – everything to which you switch your forces.

Citrine also enhances your confidence accordingly, so if you've been feeling at the back of your foot lately, turn to these crystals to help you get back on point and ready to say your piece.

Clear Quartz

Look no further than this crystal's very name to grasp its secret healing power. In many other words, Clear Quartz involves bringing clarity to everybody around you, letting you see things in the truth. Fortunately, when those truths are a bit ugly or difficult to handle, this crystal has some soothing energies which prevent you from getting too hurt.

Clear Quartz can heal the body and mind with equal fluency, but its specialty is vision – physical as well as spiritual. If you've been suffering from brain fog or have a scrambled mind because of the stress you've endured, this crystal can make things straight for you, giving you a broader perspective on what to do.

Dalmatian Jasper

Dalmatian Jasper, sweet and speckled, is a crystal of purely humorous energy. If you've forgotten the little joys of life somehow, or seem to be having fun with everything you do, this crystal will help you let your cheekier side play out.

This crystal also lets you accept with a sense of humor the obstacles that come into your life-only, the wisest spiritualists know how valuable such a thing can be in the game of life! Dalmatian Jasper gives you a spring in your step and joy in your heart, but don't worry – it's not going to leave you in the clouds, either.

Dumortierite

Everything nowadays seems like it must be immediate, and it can lead to some unreasonable expectations even for the best of us. Yet patience is a virtue, and that is what Dumortierite recognizes. Use this crystal to assist you in seeing the more significant journey that we're all on, and not sweat about the little things.

But apart from patience, this crystal also encourages peace of mind and the ability to react deftly to unforeseen life changes. This stone will also reveal the relationships around you that drag you down, and so many toxic influences in your life will expose their true colors.

Focus on Fluorite Crystal

Fluorite's striking colors make it a famous stone in its own right, but this stone's relaxing properties have made it so consistently popular. Always rising with stress and anxiety, this crystal is a welcome soothing balm for the soul.

Fluorite is a standard meditation aid, because it is necessary to reach the meditative state to achieve a state of absolute calmness and a quiet mind. However, if you had problems sleeping, you can also use it by placing it under your pillow.

Fuchsite

Many crystal healers see Fuchsite as a pillar of hard love. While it is invaluable for piercing through myths, eradicating harmful karmic patterns and otherwise tearing away everything that keeps you off, it has a straightforward and striking force.

However, the insight and information this stone can help you connect to are more valuable things than that of mollycoddle. By keeping this stone's powers in your mind, you will become someone who can recognize deceit and lies long before they can do any harm.

Garnet

Garnet is famous because it is a vibrant red color, and likewise, this crystal can awaken a passion for the red hot. However, this is directed towards love and a passion for anything else you love in life-art, work, fitness, or hobbies.

Garnet encourages you to make the most out of every day, and it can help you heal in the physical so that you have the energy and health to do just that. If your life has felt somewhat stuck in a rut, this gemstone can inspire you to shake things up positively.

Blue Goldstone

Of course, it makes sense that people who seek their fortune rely on Goldstone energies. It inspires both abundance and ambition and also has a feeling of good luck. You can't help but feel like a significant windfall is just around the corner with Goldstone in your pockets!

It is also a gem of hope that we could all do with as a society in today's climate of toxic media coverage and ever more enormous obstacles before us. Goldstone helps you find the inner spark of creativity inside you, and bring it to work to become a force for good change in the world.

Green Calcite

If you're searching for a return to harmony with nature or trying to find ways to escape big city life's chaos, Green Calcite can yield just the ticket. It has this beautiful quality of making growth a little slow – just enough to take some precious time, sit on the beach or walk through the garden.

Green Calcite assures us that; relaxation is just as important as motivation and achievement when it comes to success in life. Meditation with this crystal can also awaken you to the cycles that guide a great deal of experience, and through this process, you can understand your cyclic nature.

Hematite

Hematite's metallic shine may well serve to reinforce your steady determination, but this stone itself also strengthens your physical body. That means it can help you manage illness and injury, but it also gives you more resistance to disease and tiredness.

Hematite is a stone that focuses the mind and heart on the simple, measurable, real, and attainable things. If you find your head too much in the sky or your night-time dreams are so vivid that you wake up in amazement, this stone will offer useful grounding energy.

Jade

Crystals that are rich in history and mythology are no better than Jade. It's a connection with the Aztecs, and Ancient China is documented, and the mythology surrounding this stone has been around for many years.

The reputation Jade has for protection, inspiration, motivation, and healing is just as accurate today. It is a versatile, beautiful, and highly sought-after stone, and with age, it seems that its energies and beauty only increase.

Jade offers those willing to work with its energies wisdom and abundance, and it can open your understanding of the innate duality of life.

K2 Stone

Called from the Himalayan Mountain, K2 Stone is likewise intent on helping you ascend to new heights. It is a combination of fused stones, and its colorings are like a bright summer sky.

This stone is said to strengthen one's capacity to survive harsh living conditions. Sometimes all of the world's energies and crystals cannot change a bad situation as fast as we need it, and so we need to go through a process until it finished before we can finish it.

Similarly, in terms of physical health and healing, this crystal shows that you have to learn to live with certain medical conditions.

Kambaba Jasper

It is a crystal that speaks to one's most primitive parts and allows us to understand that such things are just part of human existence.

Of course, there is always every incentive to pursue enlightenment and still move beyond ourselves. But Kambaba Jasper will help you maintain your power and perseverance during these cycles and remind you, if things go wrong, to take it easy on yourself. After all, you are only human!

Labradorite

It seems like all the magical and ethereal colors are inside a piece of Labradorite; that you might picture swirling into shapes. This stone's many colors, especially its blues and greens, display how it brings harmony to multiple chakras, like the chakras of the throat and the heart.

This crystal amplifies the emotional powers and spiritual bonding. Meditation undertaken with this crystal is always much more vibrant, and a piece of this stone under your pillow inspires lively vivid night-time dreams.

Lapis Lazuli

Lapis Lazuli's high vibrations make it a beautiful crystal to anyone who wants to track their spiritual growth quickly. There are no real shortcuts to enlightenment, of course, but there are certainly ways to increase your receptivity to divine guidance, and this stone is one such way.

This crystal encourages clear-mindedness as well as clarity and authenticity in your correspondence. It helps you connect to higher ideas and thoughts and also to more mundane living principles and to see your physical and spiritual self as two halves of the same whole.

Leopard-Skin Jasper

The speckles and streaks that makeup Leopard Skin Jasper's distinctive colors and markings show that we all have our patterns and characteristics. This crystal and its energies help you see that you is no shame in being who you are.

But doing so, of course, means a lot of healing and growth – so, fortunately, this stone can help you with that too. It links the various points inside you, which will help you break the chains that prevent you from being at your best. But it will also provide the compassion you need to forgive yourself, and everybody else that might have wronged you along the way.

Lepidolite

Lepidolite is known as the crystal of progress but also a gem, which reminds us that it takes time to progress. It's also often painful or depends on being lost or leaving behind that which is old or obsolete.

The bigger picture gets focused as you work with Lepidolite's healing energies. It will give you the power to step back and observe the course of life from afar, as well as to take heart in the understanding that any discomforts in today's journey are only temporary.

Lepidolite helps you in all aspects of evolution, including physical transformation, meaning it is an excellent dietary aid or a new look to cultivate.

Polished Lodolite Quartz

Lodolite is a kind of quartz, with various inclusions of color and form. Sometimes these inclusions imitate underwater scenes, deserts, and gardens. Lodolite is also known as Quartz, Lodelite, and Lodalite Inclusion.

Lodolite can be used for meditation purposes. Its powerful yet soothing energies can instantly put you in a state of deep meditation. It will bring manifestation energies in your life so that you can fulfill the desires of your heart.

Malachite

Malachite is one of the most well-known of the green crystals and is a stone deeply connected to the chakra of the heart. It makes it a good companion for any cardiac journeys you may be on, even if you are searching for answers in your love life.

Malachite is for energy to tap into when you're healing from heartbreak, or otherwise looking to bring back into alignment an unbalanced heart chakra. It may also help with chest pain, breathing problems, and even circulation throughout the body.

Mookaite Jasper

Mookaite is a crystal that is connected deeply to everything physical and tangible. It means it can help you on your way to material success, but it also has grounding energies, which prevent you from becoming so lost in daydreams that you never take action.

Action is Mookaite's game name, and this stone's most significant rewards come to those who use their resources to make great strides in life or travel. If you're looking to expand your horizons, learn a new language, or explore a new world, the stone to choose from is Mookaite.

Moonstone

With its translucent appearance otherworldly texture, Moonstone crystal is always searched out by those who try to extend their dreams beyond just what is conceivable on this planet. The moon associated with tarot and astrology as well as secret feelings and hidden intentions, though not necessarily cruel ones, is often the energy associated with this crystal.

Moonstone is especially good at repairing rifts in relationships and, at the same time, inspiring new lovers to open their hearts. Moonstone can promote a worried couple's calm and serenity, but it can illuminate any flaws which prevent a romance from working out.

Mother Pearl's

Pearl's mother, also known as nacre, is a sparkling layer of material that forms the lining of many mollusks.

Mother of Pearl's resonant energies will enhance your interpersonal skills and guide you in a more effective way of expressing yourself. It is a potent stone of protection. It will bring the gentle power of the sea to heal you! It is an influential stone which will activate the chakras of your solar plexus and throat. It'll work to send out the heart's wisdom to the people around you.

Obsidian

Obsidian is a very evocative and enigmatic gem, because of its black color and overall luster. Nevertheless, as with other black crystals, protective are the principal energies at work in this stone.

When you still feel bowled over by other people's influential personalities, or otherwise have a hard time confronting boisterous people, this crystal can not only keep you safe; it can also encourage you to speak out. Obsidian is also a stone of self-reflection, though; it will coax you to explore and work on the imperfections inside you that you would otherwise not face up.

Ocean Jasper

Life can sometimes feel as unknowable as the sea, but Ocean Jasper reminds us that we can ride the currents of life accordingly, at least. It is a crystal that tells you to relax and recognize that many of the greatest journeys in life are the ones that lead to unexpected destinations.

Hold your Ocean Jasper close by when you feel depressed by your life circumstances. This crystal will help you, so to speak, reach the surface and remain afloat when you feel like the tides of your items are trying to drag you.

Onyx

Deep and mysterious, as many darker crystals are, Onyx is a protective stone. It is also a crystal that awakens your inner trust and can help you find a healthier balance of humility and self-esteem.

If you feel like people are walking all over you or have been taking advantage of your compassion for too long, Onyx might help you stand firm. If you have also been caught up in what feels like it's an impossible choice, then Onyx can help improve your decision-making capacity.

Oranges Calcite

Orange Calcite's summer sunshine feel helps activate your positivity and gives you the insight you need into the right opportunities that will come your way. When they grow, it always takes bravery to reach out to new prospects, and this crystal will help you do just that.

However, if you feel haunted by past events or can't let go of old hurt, this crystal can help heal those spiritual wounds and sever your ties with them. It'll result in a new lease of life, provided you can commit to the necessary soul work.

Peridot

Peridot is known as the crystal that radiates light and, in addition to that, a sense of positivity and abundance. It is a gem of wealth, and if you still find yourself trapped in a kind of shortage mentality, it can also help turn your thoughts around.

Peridot has healing and inspiration qualities, which make it very famous among people with creative minds and practical sides, which means that those looking for reliable solutions can embrace their approach. This stone collaborates with your heart chakra and helps you find as effective a way as possible to get a balance while helping others and looking after yourself.

Picture Jasper

Picture Jasper has a rich earthy quality that helps cultivate calming energies and general love as well as taking it slow when you need to. This crystal will help you remain steady and unshakeable in following your goals.

It is good sometimes to be a bit stubborn! Otherwise, we might easily be deterred from what we set out and do. This crystal is one of staying the path and keeping your promises.

It's also a crystal that attracts you to abundance, meaning it's popular with those who seek to boost their finances or good fortune in other areas of the world.

Pyrite

You probably know that Pyrite is often called Fool's Gold, but don't let it fool you by its comparative lack of monetary value! This crystal is an excellent companion to help you find your wealth and accept the ideas you need.

However, Pyrite often promotes self-reflection, and by spending quality time with the stone, you can come to know about your self-qualities that do not support your higher purpose. If you are trying to stop bad habits or conquer what's holding you back, Pyrite's your buddy.

Red Jasper

This stone's vibrant color is primarily associated with the root chakra-the very chakra that connects each one of us to the physical world. This crystal, however, is at a more accessible level that reminds you to take good care of yourself day by day.

Red Jasper and its energies are innately nurturing, and they encourage you to cut yourself a little slack if things go wrong or you make judgment lapses. Likewise, if you've been unwell, this stone's energies will help you get a faster recovery.

Rhodochrosite

Rhodochrosite's sweet cotton candy color is a clear example of how the crystal's energy perceives treats. While it is affordable enough, it is a stone of self-acceptance, and of remembering that we are worthy of love.

If you've been putting your interests on the back burner so long you don't know how to make yourself happy anymore, this crystal will help. It will remind you of those little things you love, and it will give you the means to communicate with them and make you just a little more confident and ready to take on the challenges of life.

Rhodonite

Interested in the long game plan, this is what helps to encourage Rhodonite. This crystal gives you insight into the cycles of life and makes you realize that you often need to plant seeds well ahead of their collection to make the most of things.

It can guide you intuitively when it comes to making investment opportunities or planning a career path, and it can also help you choose a long-term partner. However, this crystal also encourages you not to give up on life too quickly when unexpected incidents arise and stay the path.

Rhyolite

Rhyolite is a crystal that helps you to view existing circumstances from a new perspective. It's not always that easy, but this stone can help make it happen.

Equally, if your life has become a small humdrum and is boring, you can see it again with the influence of the Rhyolite vibrations.

This crystal is optimistic, but it does not encourage any illusions to pursue it. Rhyolite is an excellent crystal to see if you want the right balance in keeping it real and looking at the bright side.

Rose Quartz

Love and affection know no bounds as Rose Quartz, and its energies all too well know. This crystal is not only typical for a romance, but also of family love, career love, or even life love itself. If you have felt love, this impact is much appreciated!

This stone also inspires the emotions, such as humility and forgiveness, that go in hand with love. If you're looking to heal differing opinions, or rifts in relationships otherwise close, this crystal can help out.

Rutilated Quartz

Most faith healers and spiritually minded crystal collectors appreciate rutilated quartz because of how it can so efficiently filter negative energies out of their lives. If pessimism in everything around you overcomes you, this crystal can refresh that perspective to a more balanced one.

Yet this crystal will also help you remove your negativity as well. It can cleanse one's heart and mind, even if it occurs to be subconscious, of any resentment you hold. Many of these negative emotions will make your spiritual growth very sluggish, making this stone a helpful ally.

Selenite

The essence of illumination and light makes selenite an essential crystal for those wishing to see the spiritual reality. This crystal can help open your third-eye chakra and lead to some fascinating spiritual insights.

It is a crystal of purification, both for yourself and for your community. Many people look at putting selenite at home or in their workplace to hold negative feelings and reduce vibration energies in the background. You can be your best self by keeping the light and airy.

Serpentine

The serpentine stone works with the smaller chakras, and as such, it can help alleviate any concerns you have with the physical world-or physical intimacy.

If you are down throughout the physical realm that you're totally out of balance with your higher and spiritual self, this crystal can somehow scale. Its color helps to awaken you to nature's healing powers and how you can take better care of yourself. Serpentine is a crystal that enables many people to attract wealth in all its forms, making it a good luck charm.

Shungite

Shungite is a black stone but also one linked to countless possibilities for healing. One of the intrigues of these is the crystal's detoxifying properties, meaning poor life choices can be fought back by this stone.

For example, the crystal also allows you to stick with a healthy lifestyle overall by getting self-control. Shungite has an aspect of purity that can help you find the means for keeping things simple when you need to.

Smoky Quartz

If you've felt as if your progress in life has been obscured from sight due to negative emotions, Smoky Quartz can help heal that and overcome the pain.

Smoky Quartz crystal helps you reconnect with the wonders of living. Under this energy, every day begins to feel like a new opportunity, and the positive vibrations that you will welcome from this crystal can help you see the possibilities before you.

Smoky Quartz helps you find emotional balance, but it also brings you into greater harmony with others around you – ideal if someone's behavior has confused you lately.

Sodalie

Sodalite is, in many respects, one of the crystal world's great equalizers. If you feel so negative that you can't get yourself motivated to make changes to your life – or so inflated with good feelings that your feet never touch the ground – Sodalite helps bring everything into balance.

Sodalite, however, is also strongly associated with psychic energies, and helps adjust to your most profound intuitive insights. Because of this, Sodalite has become a trendy meditation stone, and that means you will be able to gain new insights through all these journeys into yourself.

Sunstone

Just like Sunstone, few crystals can honestly charge your creative side up. More than that, this crystal will strengthen your ideas with grounded thinking that means you don't feel stumped in how to follow them as you come up with exciting new directions to carry your life.

Better still, this is trustingly an excellent stone. Ever had a fantastic idea and gave it up because it seemed like everyone was talking it down? Sunstone will perhaps inspire you to stick a little bit more to those bright ideas. You never know what incredible progress you might make if you let yourself thrive like this!

Tiger Eye

The name is befitting, leave it to Tiger's Eye to be the stone you need to feel brave when it's time. It awakens a bolder side of you, and it does so in a not superficial way.

That's because the kind of energy that Tiger's Eye provides is self-esteem and more in-depth insight into yourself – your strengths and weaknesses. Confidence comes from just these observations, and so it is only natural that you will be braver resonate with those sides of yourself.

Tourmalinated Quartz

This distinctive stone has Tourmaline strands and streaks in the Quartz core, and in one convenient package, it also blends clarity and power. This crystal will amplify your natural energy to make your best self come true and will allow you to reflect on your needs and desires.

Through these discoveries, you'll feel encouraged with a renewed passion for following your life path. Tourmalinated Quartz allows you to be independent and know who you can count on when in a pinch.

Agate Tree

The most potent oaks can grow from the smallest of acorns, Tree Agate can help you understand how to nurture your ideas, best visions, and plans now so that they can stand the long-term test of time.

The crystal is one of healing and introspection as well. It will help you to understand any issues that have arisen in your life of love. It will also bring you into closer harmony with natural remedies and places of deep spiritual significance, away from the city thrum.

CHAPTER THREE

Uses Of Crystals

Perhaps the crystal's highest value is its use in healing. They have long been recognized for their curative effects when used in tincture preparation, for their protective features when worn as amulets and talismans, and for their ability to enhance the body's energy fields as they emit uniform vibrations. They hold the strength of living stone.

These quartzs' energy field, called piezoelectricity, is a significant contributor to our communications systems. Computers, sonar, radio stations, and watches? 'All use this fantastic and constant, undeviating energy field. The piezo-electric property of crystals means that they are capable of holding an electric charge. Because of this quality, these minerals amplify healing meditation, which in turn accelerates the process. Quartz is the most economical supply of this energy.

Crystals store and conduct energy; they can absorb one type of energy and emit it again when squeezed, cooled, or heated. Quartz crystal absorbs both the magnetism from the Earth's core and the radiation from Sun, and then emits that energy. Kirlian photography has documented this energy emission, which appears in photographs as a white-light aura radiating from a blue star center.

The vibration happens quickly, within a few moments of holding a crystal or gemstone in hand. Crystal energy travels through and penetrates all matter, including into human cells. Crystal energy transfer has a magnetic polarity similar to the normal aura polarity used in the laying on of hands. The unique ability to balance and interact with aura energy makes a crystal a powerful healing device.

When you start working with crystals, an exciting phenomenon happens for whatever reason. You will begin to become aware of the energy or force that is greater than what you currently contain. This force is called your Higher Self, and it includes "what you can become." It is your perfected self. Quartz crystals can help you tap into this higher dimension of yourself in their wonderfully helpful way.

A kind act is relative to crystal quartz . It helps to form a connection between you and a person. It helps you to communicate with that person, psychologically. It's also a fantastic way for someone to send healing energies, especially if you both have similar crystals. A crystal gift instils a positive effect on the recipient.

Crystals in Healing

Noted healers have shown that crystals can accelerate the healing of bones and wounds, relieve pain, and bring catastrophic disease into remission. Although some say there are no powers at all in the crystal because it is a neutral object, its inner structure showcases a state of perfection and equilibrium. Once a crystal is cut to the correct form, and the human mind enters into a relationship with its architectural excellence, the jewel creates a vibration that enhances and amplifies the healer's mind's powers. Like a laser, it radiates power in a consistent, highly concentrated form, and this energy can transmit into objects or individuals.

When people become emotionally distressed, their subtle-energy body forms a weakness, and disease may follow soon. A healer can help liberate negative patterns in the energy body with a properly tuned crystal, allowing the physical body to get to a state of wholeness.

When healers lovingly attune their minds to a crystal, they are one with the Divine Spirit, which has engraved their consciousness in that structure's precise, geometric shape.

Healers use crystals because the stone is the most perfectly organized natural state of matter. It is precise, regular, and free of flaws and impurities. When people are in tune with crystal perfection, they will make themselves beautiful.

One method of crystal healing is to lovingly tune in to the crystal's energy field, transmitting the energy into the crystal, interacting in harmony with the crystal. When you (the healer) feel charged with the crystal, scan the person's body, being sensitive to places of apparent imbalance where healing energies are to be focused. A brilliant focal point is the heart chakra, where intuitively sensed problems could bring to awareness through visualization. Then snap the crystal-like a whip-crack (by flicking the wrist and gripping the crystal by the hand), releasing the tension that was held in the subtle body.

The crystal can take the feeling for love in the healer's heart and amplify it so that a concentrated stream of energy can be remitted from the crystal for healing use. This enhanced energy field will help individuals dislodge inhibitions that obstruct the flow for their higher life energies.

The crystal operates just the same way a laser does: it takes and focuses dispersed energy rays. It makes the energy field coherent and unidirectional to produce a tremendous force. When combining with love, the crystal unites the mental energies. It puts these energies into a sequence, precisely in line with the person's life energies seeking healing, and then amplifies them for healing.

For the crystal's effectiveness, the rational mind must be turned off, so that you can enter a meditative state of the right-brain and intuitively adjust to the energies focused by the crystal transmitter.

There are many uses of crystal healing methods. Maybe the best advice to follow would be to listen to your intuition. Use what suits you best. Focus on yourself and everyone around you. Meditate and listen to what is gently suggested by the voice within you.

The general size of the crystal used for healing may fit in the palm of your hand comfortably. Its dimensions are not as crucial as their feeling or essence. There's no need to have a big piece of quartz; in most cases, a small portion would suffice.

Some potential healing methods are to place crystals or gemstones at the seven key points of the chakra. Place a crystal wherever pain or discomfort is present on the body. A gem can be kept closer to the source of pain and rotated in motion in the clockwise direction to draw the issue out. Snap the crystal to get rid of vibrations unwelcomed. For the energy to be balanced, single crystals can be placed in palms of the hands.

Crystals are excellent biofeedback tools, and they work well with creative visualization for changes in mood and body. Hold a crystal in your left hand when feeling cold or chilled, and draw warmth. Do this in a deep breathing meditation of color, pulling in energy. "Visualized as red" through the left side of the body, a circuit running through the body releases it to the Earth or sky from the right side. Continue to do so for a few minutes until you feel warm. It also works in blue for cooling.

Draw yellow in the same way for cheering; deep violet or indigo for calming. It can increase or lower body metabolism and heart rate, an impact already familiar to those who have used it for deep respiration.

Use crystals to amplify and reinforce what is achievable as visualizations, affirmations, and rituals; Use a gem in the left hand usually to receive energy and on the right side to transmit it, but in some cases, this could be the opposite. Experiment and find out what works best.

Crystals will virtually magically alleviate pain. Hold a crystal in your left hand in another self-healing exercise, feel the energy polarity built from it, gently place the right side on a pain area, and hold it there. The pain usually dissolves within half an hour.

Another method recommends setting the crystal directly on the area of pain, holding it flat with the thumb in the palm, or holding it between the fingers, pointing downwards. The pain goes away when you remove the crystal.

Crystals can be used effectively in reading the aura and in healing the character. Hold a crystal in whatever hand feels right, and scan the person's atmosphere from the head to the toes. Feel thirst, tingles, cold, resistance. Rotate the crystal counter clockwise when you encounter these, and touch the tip to the area. It stirs up the aura. A motion in the clockwise direction takes out energy. After going down the person's forehead and back, brush the atmosphere down to cleanse and seal the chakras.

Different Ways of Using Crystals

Crystals were admired for centuries for their scientific, healing, and spiritual qualities. The wide variety of ways crystals can be used is astonishing, from powering a calculator to alleviating pain.

Solar Cells

Solar cells are among the essential uses of crystals. Solar cells provide power to various devices, from calculators to space vehicles. The solar cell generates energy, called photovoltaic energy, using silicone (based on a tetragon crystal).

Transistors

Made from semi-conductors that are based on the same types of materials and crystals as solar cells, transistors can regulate electron flow, detect and amplify radio signals and therefore act as digital "switches." Note: transistor radios make use of crystals.

Liquid Crystals

From heat and electricity to mechanics and magnetism, this precise substance made from crystals can use various means. For example, wristwatches and certain clock types use liquid crystals, just like some pocket calculators do.

Spiritual Crystals

Different types of crystals have far been thought to confer certain traits or qualities on those who use them, helping them to gain access to some emotions. Accordingly, amethyst crystals are used to reduce anger and impatience. Others include aquamarine to release fear, carnelian to build confidence, coral to enhance emotions: diamonds to improve prosperity; emeralds to alleviate stress and insomnia, and sapphire to restore calmness and equilibrium.

Medicinal Crystals

Many new-age medical practitioners, in addition to their supposed spiritual benefits, assert the existence and other uses of some crystals facilitate various kinds of medical benefits. These benefits include: amethyst to treat headaches or unbalanced blood sugar; aquamarine to regulate the immune system, cardiac and lymph nodes; carnelian to help with energy, reproductive system, and menstrual cramps; citrine to cleanse spleen, kidneys, and liver; coral to help regenerate metabolism, spine, and tissue; emeralds to help with thymus and childbirth; jade to help cleanse spleen, etc.

Industrial Uses of Crystals

Early civilizations used quartz, garnet, diamonds, and other crystals like crystal sands as abrasives to create blocks of stone and rock, fashion ornamentation and jewelry, and to create specialized gravures. Science began mineral synthesis and the synthetic growth of crystals in the laboratory during the late 19th century. Synthetic gems proved to be more abrasive than their natural counterparts, being more reliable, cheaper, and easier to obtain, in many industries, synthetic crystals quickly found a healthy market.

Diamond Crystals and Dust for Cutting

The diamond bits are used for cutting stone blocks and ornamental stones in industrial saws and ropes. Diamond-studded drill bits are now used as oil well drills. Jewelers and lapidary artisans use diamond-loaded saws, diamond-loaded copper laps, and diamond polishing powder, mainly for hard-wearing.

Watches and Semiconductors

In the watch industry, synthetic quartz, ruby, and sapphire are all used. Rolex watch glass is manufactured from synthetic sapphire, which is scratch-resistant and colorless. Synthetic ruby has been used in watches and other mechanical instruments for producing reliable bearings. Synthetic quartz crystal controls the time, using a silicon chip. Pure quartz sand is used for making silicon metal, a semi-conductor that has been used in creating transistors and microelectronics production, integrated circuits, and the silicon chip.

Ruby Laser

This red-light beam was invented in 1960 and produced an intense light with minimal divergence; it has multiple applications in the industry. It can be used in CD players and long-distance telephones, surveying, and microchirurgy as well. Professors at the college and others find the tiny ruby laser pointer beneficial in their lectures. High-energy lasers can cut diamonds through steel plates and drill holes.

How to Protect Yourself with Crystals

But first, let us get on the same page about what our lives mean by "protection." According to Sadie Kadlec, Maha Rose Center for Healing's crystal specialist and intuitive healer, the notion of security being a barrier to stopping external powers (like other people or even bad energy) from reaching our domain is seriously flawed. "The real idea of protection is to find strength, stability, and support within you to be vulnerable, and to trust the world around you so there's no need to have that shield," she says. So basically, don't expect to utilize crystals as a literal protective armor that will keep all the woes in life from harming you potentially. Instead, work to embrace your inner self-confidence and sense of self, as doing so can help you find protective elements that you already inherently possess. Then, the crystals will raise the positive vibes. The best way to use stones for defense is by meditating and keeping them with you (or, if you are Miranda Kerr, sleeping with one under your pillow) as a reminder of your purpose, honesty and inner power. Obviously, crystals aren't going to solve it all, but some, particularly the following seven, will help you achieve a changed mind set and a boosted mood. Here's what Kadlec has got to say about the particular ways that every stone can work for you.

1. Fluorite

"[Protection] is about opening the heart through that cycle and finding strength in oneself," Kadlec says. Fluorite creates clarity and openness by being able to express boundaries in a manner other people can honor. During meditation, put the stone on your heart chakra to align certain energies to banish negative thought patterns from your life.

2. Kyanite

Compassionate contact encourages trust and stability in your relationships — two issues that are of prime importance to defense. For this, Kadlec says kyanite is a powerful stone, and is also associated with the chakra of the throat which governs communication. "Kyanite lets our inner truth come up and be heard," she says. "It also places us in a position to receive and hear from others." Expressing yourself creates a sense of security, so look to this stone the next time you need to tackle a tough convoy that makes you feel nervous and vulnerable.

3. Black tourmaline

Grounding stones such as black tourmaline also serve as power players for defense. Kadlec says this one is connected with the chakra of the solar plexus, where a little bolstering is sometimes required. She says that black tourmaline can absorb threatening energy and transmute it to non-threatening things. The stone will help you see circumstances within yourself or others more clearly away from negative factors, and how to respond compassionately.

Often, we feel like we're challenged because we're uncomfortable about ourselves," "We responding from that position and that's when we start creating walls that we think we need to build trust." Black tourmaline can flip these bad vibes on their heads.

4. Pyrite and citrine

Although historically these stones are not synonymous with defense, pyrite and citrine are excellent at helping us find structure. "They're about our intention's clarity — who we are, and how we can make it happen for ourselves."

So instead of always carrying the weight of the opinions and aspirations of the people, take the course of what is best for you and you alone, but without being combative. This binds back to that new and improved protection definition that is rooted in inner strength, stability, and safety.

5. Carnelian

Ready for a pep talk that will boost confidence? Great, because it is really a common factor in whether or not we feel safe and protected. "Carnelian connects us to our courage, it's where we do what's right for ourselves so that we don't silently accept what doesn't work for us." Living courageously gives us confidence and drives us to make decisions that serve us rather than reeling back in fear.

6. Malachite

Stones such as malachite can help open our hearts and address fear in the first place, removing the need to feel safe. Crystals that pull in synchronicity and abundance help to place us in the right circumstances at the right moment, It's also a powerful one to convey appreciation rather than feel overwhelmed by the race to build a bigger wall to create more room between you and your reality. And honestly, we could all use that kind of energy a little bit more in our lives.

Different types of Healing Crystals
Clear quartz

This white crystal is often considered a "master healer." It's said that by absorbing, storing, releasing and regulating it, it amplifies energy. It's said to help memory and concentration too. Physically, it's claimed that clear crystals help stimulate the immune system and balance your whole body. Often this stone is paired with others such as rose quartz to help and enhance their abilities.

Rose quartz

This pink stone is all about love, just as the color might suggest. This is said to help restore trust and harmony in all sorts of relationships while at the same time strengthening their close relations. It is also claimed to assist in providing comfort and calm in times of grief.

And it's not just about other people. Rose quartz is also said to promote love, loyalty, confidence and value within one's self — something that we could all use in present day and age.

Jasper

This smooth crystal is the "supreme nurturer." It is said to inspire the spirit and help you during times of stress by training you to "stand up" entirely. It is said to shield you from and absorb negative vibes while encouraging confidence, fast thinking and trust. Those are characteristics that are of particular benefit when coping with critical problems — which is just what this stone is used for.

Obsidian

It is said that an intense protective stone, obsidian, helps to form a shield against physical and emotional negativity. It is also said to help you get rid of emotional blockage and promote strength, clarity and compassion qualities to help you find your true sense of self. It may help digestion and detoxification for your physical body, while potentially helping to reduce pain and cramps.

Citrine

Take the citrine to every aspect of your life with laughter, wonder and excitement. It's said to help you remove negative traits like fear from your life, which in effect help promote happiness, comfort, inspiration which lead to clarity. It's also believed to improve the standard of mindfulness, such as creativity and concentration.

Turquoise

This blue crystal has powers believed to help the mind, body, and soul recover. In general, it's seen as a charm of good luck that can help balance your emotions while finding your spiritual groundings. When it comes to body, the respiratory, skeletal, and immune system are said to benefit.

Tiger's eye

If you need a boost in strength or inspiration, the golden stone could be for you. It's said to help get rid of terror, anxiety and self-doubt in your mind and body. It can be perfect for career goals, or even heart problems. Also, the eye of Tiger is said to help guide you towards harmony and balance to help you make clear, conscious decisions.

Amethyst

It is said that this purple stone is highly defensive, curative and purifying. It's believed that it can help rid the mind of negative thoughts and put modesty, honesty and spiritual wisdom into being. It's known to help encourage sobriety too. Sleep is another claimed advantage of this stone, from supposedly helping in relief from insomnia to understanding dreams. Physically, it is said to boost the production of hormones, cleanse the blood and relieve pain and stress.

Moonstone

Known for "new beginnings," it's said that moonstone encourages inner growth and energy. This stone is supposed to soothe those uncomfortable feelings of stress and instability when starting fresh so that you can move forward successfully. It's also said to encourage positive thought, insight and motivation while at the same time bringing wealth and prosperity.

Bloodstone

This powerful Stone of Healing lives up to its name. Bloodstone is claimed to also help cleanse the blood by extracting bad energy from the environment and improving circulation. In a mindful way, it fosters selflessness, imagination and idealism thus enabling you to live in the present moment. It's also said that it will help you get rid of irritability, aggressiveness and impatient feelings too.

Sapphire

The blue stone is one of royalty and wisdom. It's said that while opening the mind to accept beauty and intuition it can attract prosperity, happiness and peace. As far as the physical health is concerned, this stone is also claimed to help cure eye problems, cellular levels and blood disorders while also relieving depression, anxiety and insomnia.

Ruby

A red standout, this stone helps to restore the energy and vitality levels. This can help in things like sensuality, sex, and intellect improvement. It's also said to help add self-awareness to one's mind and realize reality. In ancient times rubies were used to help remove toxins from the blood and to improve the circulatory system as a whole.

How to Care for your Crystal

When you bring home your crystal for the first time, you're going to want to clean up any negativity it may have gathered. This can be kept under cold, flowing water from a tap, or rinsed in a natural water stream. Sure, the water is cold, not hot or warm, either way.

Add the cleanse or burn sage with a bit of sea salt to really help it get rid of unwanted energies. You may also leave it to dry in sunlight or full moon light to let the light pass through.

However, it is not just about their physical care. In order for crystals to work their magic, you must mentally remove the negative energy or skepticism you might have about their abilities. It is important that what they can do for you is respected.

Crystal accessories

Crystals can have the main benefit of their healing abilities. But if we're perfectly honest, then they're very beautiful too. So, it's no surprise people make tons of accessories like jewelry or home decorations out of them. The crystals will not only look nice, they will never hurt anyone while keeping good energy around.

Prayer beads

Crystal beads of prayer are worn against the heart to inspire all sorts of positive feelings, be they hope, courage or peace. They are a great way for anyone to carry about crystal healing powers.

Jewelry

Jewelry is another great way to embed the capabilities of a crystal. Not to mention, it also lets you show off the beauty of each stone.

Coasters

These stunning coasters are made from genuine Brazilian gemstones. In this household element, the agate stone will help foster peace and harmony within the home. These are ideal for those who would like to bring good energies to their homes.

Sex toys

These crystal sex toys blend their energies with your sexual energy to help deliver pure, sexual pleasure. They're fantastic tools to help those who've been in a sexual rut break free.

Pipes

Believe it or not, even crystal-made hand pipes can make you smoke. They are soft, easy to use and robust. This makes them a great gift to anyone who treats a health condition using medical marijuana.

Water bottles

Trendy water bottles are as trendy now as crystals, so it's no surprise that the two have merged into one. A "gem pod" sits in the bottom of these elegant glass bottles. It's said to encourage everything from health to elegance to harmony. This is a perfect accessory for making your next yoga practice come true.

If you are skeptical about these healing crystals already, then they probably won't do you any good. They're unlikely to harm you in anyway. While there is no conclusive evidence for crystals, this has not stopped people from trying them.

The key to achieving the positive qualities these beautiful stones can offer is an open mind. Whether it's good energy you want or specific healing powers overall, there's nothing wrong with giving an honest try to crystals. Who knows maybe you'll be pleasantly shocked.

CHAPTER FOUR

Crystal Combinations

I was asked what crystals work and what gems shouldn't be added. I haven't experienced a situation where crystals didn't fit together well, but there are some things I keep in mind when mixing crystals.

Opposing Energies and Too Much

Typically, I feel crystals work well together, but be careful of crystals that may have an opposing impact for energy like Carnelian, versus Blue Lace Agate or other soothing stones. The combination of two crystals with a very high vibration or powerful energy can be a specific concern for different people. For example, some may consider the combination of Moldavite and Phenacite overwhelming. Standard results such as lepidolite and lithium quartz are very calming and contain lithium, but be aware that it could also be too much of one thing.

Intention, Intuition, Simplicity

What does it mean to you? What is it you're trying to do? Fill your intentions up like:

Healing (Green Aventurine), bones (Calcite), or Citrine for problems with the stomach.

Use your instincts because that's your compass. It is. I know everybody's saying this, but it's the truth!

Please keep it simple before combining, and know-how crystals work for you individually. We see these massive, complicated grids of crystals on social media. For sure, they are stunning, but please don't feel overwhelmed by them. Smaller, less costly, or fancy jewels will accomplish the same goals. It isn't about the bling. It's about your wishes!

Color

Color is a decent starting point, but there is a lot more to work with crystals than the frequency of color alone. You may use a color wheel to look like a reference to competing colors. It does work out often, though. I use Red Jasper, Green Aventurine or Malachite, or other red crystals. They oppose colors, but, in some circumstances, they work.

Crystal Structure

It may sound boring and all geo-geeky, I know, but bear with me. The crystal structure can help you determine how crystals are combined.

Cubic (or isometric) system of crystals, are based on a square structure within -- Pyrite, Gold, Garnet, Magnetite, Fluorite, Diamond.

Hexagonal Crystals rely on an inner hexagonal (6-faced) structure – Beryl, Emerald, Apatite, Morganite, Aquamarine, and Sugilite.

Trigonal system of crystals (Rhombohedral system) are based on an inner triangular structure - Calcite, Quartz, agate, aventurine, jasper, hematite, carnelian,

Calcite
A family of crystals

I love to combine the crystals based on their family of gems. The Quartz family, for example, Clear Quartz, Rose Quartz, Smokey Quartz, Citrine, Amethyst, etc. Many of these Agates, Calcite, Jaspers, Tourmalines, etc. can be added. Jaspers, agates, and quartz all fit well together too.

The Elements

Working with Gems in terms of the elements is not a field in which I am overly educated, but more work on this is something to be done. Several different cultures and philosophies are leading to contradictory facts, but the elements are Earth, Air, Fire, Water, and Spirit, for example.

Air / Wind Stones -Amethyst, Fluorite, Selenite, Labradorite, Sugilite.

Fire Stones-Amber, Carnelian, Citrine, Sunstone, Fire Agate, Fire Opal, Red Jasper.

Sunstone

Earth Stones-Agate, Jade, Halite, Hematite, Jasper, Gold, Onyx, Obsidian, Garnet, Pyrite, Black Tourmaline.

Water Stones-Amethyst, Aquamarine, Moonstone, Agate, Blue Bracelet, Celestite, Chalcedon, Rose Quartz, Chrysocolla, Sea Salt, Selenite, Pearl, Larimar.

Spirit / Naisha Ashian has Storm as an element, so it varies from one to another: Apophyllite, Danburite, Diamond, Phenacite, Clear Quartz.

General guidelines: Combine air with gas and water with earth. In contrast, it might not be a great combo to combine (FIRE) - Carnelian / Citrine and (WATER) - Blue Lace Agate.

Naisha Ahsian Crystal Ally Cards is an excellent resource for learning about the elements and the crystals.

Some of My Favorite Combos

Power, inspiration, strength, control, getting things done: Carnelian and citrine. Citrine is an excellent stone to use by breaking them up and dissipating them to counter toxic energy of any sort. Clearing unnecessary energies off the atmosphere is beneficial. Citrine is a glad stone. It can bring joy to the person carrying it or wearing it. It can relieve depression, self-doubt, rage, and irrational mood swings, due to its removal of negative energy and bringing positivity. Citrine is used to reduce tendencies toward self-destruction. Citrine helps to overcome emotional traumas and grief that can lead to these self-destructive emotional issues. Carnelian wearing can boost vitality and will, providing the energy needed when reaching new projects and dreams. On the home front, Carnelian is useful to keep on hand to prevent accidents, especially for the do-it-yourselfer. It is used against theft, fire, and storm damage to the home. Mentally, Carnelian focuses on analytical skills and improves reflection by allowing for deeper concentration and not interrupting thoughts. Carnelian helps make choices by keeping us focused on the here and now and not past experiences. Carnelian calms you down when angry and grounds you while keeping you conscious of the Universe's unconditional Love. Carnelian promotes commitment and initiative. Carnelian has a lot of life force, stimulating metabolism and providing the organs and tissues with good blood supply. It influences both sexes' reproductive organs, and increases fertility and overcomes frigidity and impotence. It helps with symptoms of menstruation and menopause and may assist in vitro and artificial insemination.

Readings: labradorite, celestine, danburite. These healing crystal can be great to calm down and to balance. Some people who used this crystal have stated that it also helps them remember their dreams. Additionally, the Celestine crystal will help to give your body clarity and calm. The Celestine crystal can be particularly useful for those with the following signs of the zodiac: Gemini. This crystal of healing reflects faith, happiness, and dreams. Its advantages and properties also include fostering divinity, fostering mental and physical harmony, enhancing spiritual contact, enhancing one's natural intuition, and, ultimately, balancing one's crown chakra. Labradorite Crystal is a magic stone, which awakens mystical and magical abilities and psychic powers within you. They possess a profoundly felt resonance within them that is very strong. They can be used to bring positive changes to your life, and their vibration also carries a significant degree of negative security, so they can't be used for ill will. These crystals have many attributes that make them crystals that may be used by many people. It is a stone whose energy is evident to the consumer because it seems to be working so hard.

Sleeping: Amethyst, Rose Quartz, and Blue Lace Agate sometimes. The amethyst and rose quartz crystal pair were not only ordinary on Stevens Universe but when combined, become the path of physical to spiritual energy. My mom came to tears as I gifted an amethyst necklace matched with a rose quartz necklace. "You put together the sweetest of my crystals. Perfect birthday with a baby present!" I swear that I wear turquoise and that I write nothing but the truth!

Stress / Anxiety: Quartz lithium, Lepidolite, Quartz rose. We feel that self-love is a superpower at this little crystal shop and the real foundation of all true personal power. The pink Rose Quartz is commonly regarded as the stone of unconditional love and is said to attract enjoyment in all forms. It is especially suitable for the promotion of emotional harmony and self-love.

When we're tired, it can be hard to remember to take care of ourselves. Keeping a piece of Rose Quartz where we can see it, like at a nightstand or next to the bath, can act as a powerful visual reminder to take a little "me time" every day – even if it's only two quiet minutes spent alone, breathing deeply and not staring at a phone. Lepidolite can help us overcome depression by encouraging self-love and trust. The gentle lilac-rose lepidolite soothes the nervous system. One of the most potent crystals for relieving stress and anxiety is this beautiful lilac stone. It contains lithium, which is naturally used in anti-anxiety medicines. It gives calm at stressful times when we feel stressed or excessively concerned emotionally. It can dissipate any form of negativity too.

Fear/bad dreams: Smokey Quartz and Tourmaline black. When you're dealing with nightmares, protecting yourself from the negative factors that cause them is crucial. Smokey quartz excels here. Smokey quartz neutralizes harmful energy from the Crown Chakra right down to the Root Chakra with its high vibrational strength. It releases anxiety and fills you with optimistic thoughts. Black Tourmaline is a robust calming stone, electric in nature, offering a bond between earth and the human spirit. It's excellent at absorbing and repelling negativity. The rock promotes a sense of power and confidence in oneself, enabling a brighter, more objective view of the world. It also protects against pollutants from the environment and radiation.

Concentration / Focus: Fluorite and Amethyst. Focusing is crucial to your success. Whether you wish to improve in your career, learn new skills, be a better parent, or any other endeavor, this is true. If your mind wanders, you make mistakes, and the quality of your work suffers. Problem-solving becomes more laborious, and a lack of progress can be frustrating. It is where crystals really can be of help. Crystals enhance your mental processes by working through the upper chakras to give you a sense of calmness. The effect is higher concentration and attention.

Ancient wisdom: Lemurians, Quartz lamps, Quartz Tibetans.

Hiking: Jasper Rainforest, Labradorite, Aquamarine. Such crystals are useful in avoiding procrastination. Holding them on your body will help you do some of the tasks you avoided. It also has an energy that can boost your creativity, a bonus. Green Rhyolite's vibration of happiness and joy becomes a stream of positive feelings that will flow throughout your life. It is an excellent stone to help your overall self-esteem. Ths is because it resonates within the solar plexus, also known as the chakra of personal power.

General: Citrine or Pyrite, Black tourmaline or Magnetite, Quartz. Manifesting can be a reliable way to make your wishes come true. Yet when you suffer from mental and physical blockages, it may not be easy to demonstrate. Crystals are an excellent tool for overcoming such blockages. You can also balance your Chakras with the right healing crystals, amplify your intention, and disperse negativity. That provides the best opportunities to reflect and manifest.

• Grounding: Red Jasper, Black Tourmaline, and Lodestone or Hematite. These stones allow you to live in the present moment. Place the crystals around your prone body in an inverted triangle-from the waist level to under your feet. Flint, smokey quartz, magnesite, charoite, hematite, or any other grounding crystals may be used. Lay there for about half an hour, and let Earth connect. Please choose one of the crystals from your grid and then carry it with you to help you stay connected.

Pain: Malachite, and any pain. I use Smokey Quartz or Black Onyx with the Malachite, for example, if my foot hurts. I use Black Tourmaline and Malachite, or Amethyst and Malachite, if my head hurts.

Sadness: Jasper Yellow, and Jasper Fancy. This stone will give you powerful grounding energies, which will make you feel calm and serene even during stressful times. Yellow Jasper infuses you with feelings of completeness and wholeness. Its powers should work for the integration of all facets of your life.

Love: Rose quartz, Green Aventurine, or Green Tourmaline. A crystal pendulum in your chakra points for detecting and fixing energy shortages and excess rose quartz, and amethyst operates on heart and crown chakra by itself. It binds your heart to your guardian angels and your spirit.

Moonstone Crystal: Combination of Moonstone and Rose Quartz. An ethereal mixture of love and chakra synchronicity, rose quartz, and moonstone makes you a beautiful divine human. For young brides, the adularescence of moonstone makes it a fertile stone, and rose quartz holds the marriage rooted in love. Yet another gem pairing together for love, moonstone and rose quartz can awaken both your psychic powers and deep-seated emotions.

Cold: Moss Agate for the immune system, Blue Lace Agate for the throat, and occasionally Carnelian for the vitality. Perfect for sinus, cough, mucous infections, lymph node swelling, post-nasal drip, fevers reduction. Excellent for sore throats, tonsillitis, laryngitis, etc. For diseases like tonsillitis, however, be sure to seek proper medical treatment such as antibiotics, since no crystal will eliminate it. However, when held on the throat, Blue Lace Agate may help to ease some of the pain.

Whack hormones: Various colored moonstones. Moonstone, beautiful stone for fertility, pregnancy, childbirth, and all motherhood related things (In fact, it's referred to as "the stone of motherhood"). This creamy gem is thought to balance female hormones and is an immensely strong crystal to relieve stress, increase intuition, and stabilize emotions. If you ever wanted to improve your psychic powers, it's the stone to hold on hand. Meditate any time you feel off-kilter in any way with this incredibly powerful gem.

Skin: Quartz pink and Aventurine green. There's nothing better than a bit of warmth and love to fill up life, and that's where green aventurine and rose quartz gel together well. Get your crystal pairing with rose quartz and aventurine crystal pairings to attract love. Persephone, the mighty spring goddess, and Tara the night goddess make green Aventurine the stone for women with dreams and aspirations ahead of them. When combined with the potent energies of rose quartz, it brings together the strength of Aphrodite, the goddess of love and Venus. It is the ultimate crystal love potion to draw in your true love.

Meditation: Danburite, Auralite, Lazuli Lapis, Celestite, Lemurian, Phenacite, Selenite, Apophyllite, Herkimer Diamonds, Labradorite, Transparent Quartz combos. These are among the most calming crystals for meditation work. Their ethereal quality leads to a higher level of wisdom to your practice, protecting your energy field in the process. During meditation, the pure white vibration is amplified, and your crown and higher chakras open. It gives you clarity of mind, goddess consciousness, and accurate psychic insights. Before meditating, use a selenite wand to cleanse your body of negative energies and blocks of power. Then allow the high-frequency vibrations of selenite to flow through you, balancing the energy created via your practice.

The Benefits of Crystals

There are many crystals you've probably heard of all along in your life. Some common crystals include quartz, amethyst, rose quartz, citrine, and more. What makes every crystal special is that they are all capable of healing and tending to our individual needs. Sometimes it can be challenging, talking about the benefits of crystals because there is a lot of skepticism that gathers around whether or not they do as claimed. As someone who has used crystals for years, I can guarantee they can do countless wonders for your mental and physical health if you give your heart and soul up. I want you to know some of the benefits of crystals that I experienced as a way of encouraging you to experience them.

Provides a Boost of Energy

We need to have enough energy to get through busy days and to stay productive all the time. Bloodstone is a mineral that helps remove everything that occupies our mind and prevents us from getting positive thoughts. As a result, we'll feel more excited and optimistic about taking on our days with this crystal.

Allows Us to Give and Acquire Love

Uniting and spreading love together is something that I truly believe will change this world. With more respect, we can make the world a much better place in this life. Rose quartz is an excellent crystal for awakening our hearts to love giving and receiving. This crystal helps us to walk away from the things in the past that hurt us and to move ahead and live a beautiful life.

Relieves Anxiety and Stress

It is essential to find ways that work best for you to alleviate any anxiety and stress that may affect your mental, physical, and spiritual health in life. Going about with my blue lace agate crystal is one of my go-to ways of doing this. Whenever I feel an intense sense of anxiety or tension, I take this crystal with me everywhere I go and even incorporate it into my practices in mediation. This crystal emits calm, soothing energy that will always make my mind more relaxed.

Boosts Creativity

As someone who relies heavily on imagination to carry out my dreams and plans, I am often cranking out creative ideas daily that can be incredibly challenging. I love keeping my carnelian stone with me to help with this. Just looking at the stone lets my mind reveal its best ideas. The colors emit most of the positive energy and foster the trust you need to take pride in your thoughts and share them with others.

Are you fascinated by crystals, and do you regularly use them in your daily lives? I'd love to hear about your favorites and how they helped you!

The Health Benefits of Crystals

Halotherapy, also known as salt therapy, has existed for over 150 years. It dates back to Eastern Europe's salt mines and caves, where a Polish doctor called Feliks Boczowski found salt miners had fewer respiratory problems than the general population, which he attributed to repeated inhalation of salt particles. In the 1950s, Eastern European doctors started simulating conditions found within salt caves to give patients as a method of respiratory therapy. A lot of wellness centers and spas in the U.S. these days often integrate salt therapy into their activities.

"Salting therapy works at many levels," says Diana Leone, owner of Pasadena's The Salt Studio. "Healing with salt in the purest form relies on its natural antimicrobial properties to purify, draw moisture, and reduce inflammation. The fine particles of pure sodium chloride can be inhaled down into the lungs and absorbed through the pores. They help reduce the uncomfortable inflammation of asthma, allergies, and skin conditions and gently extract extra moisture and pollutants from the lungs."

We experience invisible charged particles in the air daily, called positive and negative ions. Positive ions are formed by high winds, pollution, dust, and humidity and have been shown to have adverse effects on the body when excessively exposed to them. Some of these have fatigue, asthma, depression, and irritability. On the other hand, negative ions are abundant in nature — especially in forests, at the beach, and around waterfalls — and are reported to have a positive effect on one's health, mood, and energy levels.

Being in a salt room provides an area rich in negative ions, making it extremely easy to rest and detoxify your body from the unnatural positive ions that occur every day. It results in a chance to return to the natural state, recharge, and a more alert yet relaxed feeling emerging. Serotonin also boosts negative ions so that we can feel lighter and happier.

The walls are made of pure salt from the sea, and the Himalayan salt lamps are placed as a secondary form of salt therapy throughout. Although the salt lamps' effects are not as powerful, they emit negative ions and make a great addition to one's bedroom, workplace, or other living space, contributing to a negative-ion atmosphere and encouraging relaxation. It's great for both kids and pregnant women too. I recommend visiting one anywhere for maintenance from twice a week to treat a symptom or condition once a month. There is a way for all to incorporate salt therapy into their lives for regular use as a treatment or occasional relaxation.

Guide to Healing Crystals

Crystals have been used as sources of healing power throughout history; Each crystal has its properties associated with helping balance the body and manifests one's intentions. They may be worn as jewelry, held in a bag, or displayed in their homes or offices. Here are guidelines to some of the most common crystals and their advantages.

Amethyst

It helps to heal mental and physical problems, relieves stress, and avoids nightmares.

Black Tourmaline

Protects against lousy energy; prevents one's energy from draining away.

Citrine

Channels the sun's optimistic energies to achieve goals; fosters joy, good health, wealth, and creativeness.

Clear Quartz

Used for purifying and re-energizing other crystals, counteracts toxic energy.

Labradorite

They clear one's aura, offering security, and helping to overcome negative feelings.

Rose Quartz

Magnifying feelings of self-love and other people's unconditional love; helps heal one from grief, trauma, or a broken heart.

Emotional Effects of Healing Crystals

Why do gemstones make you feel emotional? Can I think through vibe or aura from the power of gemstones? Why do I feel like I fall on gemstones when I touch them? Find the secrets of gem Emotional Effects!

Shaky

Shakiness happens when you feel overwhelmed with pain. When handling overpowering gemstones, the same shakiness is observed. For instance, if you are sad or troubled while holding a twin rose quartz stone, you might tremble and quiver with its higher heart powers.

Irritated

If you are suddenly pissed off when walking in the crystal shop by a crystal, it has to be a clash with your aura or astral chart energies. If you are a criminal or heavy sinner, malachite can drive you insane, it is merely part of healing.

Angry

Another emotional impact of crystal healing on the psyche is rage. If using a red jasper stone, and you feel angry, your basal chakra is unbalanced. For efficient removal, you need to eject the negativity curdled inside of you with a crystal pendulum. The sacral chakra is targeted.

Falling into Earth

A grounding effect of root and crown chakra stones can be excellent at certain times when you feel like you're sinking through the earth. Soiling the excess resources also means pouring them into the ground. Be careful when handling grounding stones if you feel puzzled.

Floating

You may feel you are floating because of the gemstones' dissociative effects. It doesn't happen with every healing stone, but mostly with the highest or lowest chakra stones. The floating sensation can be a disorienting signal to you.

CHAPTER FIVE

Chromotherapy

Chromotherapy, sometimes referred to as color therapy, is an alternative medicine method considered by pseudoscience. Chromotherapists claim to have the ability to use light in the form of color to restore "power" that is missing in a person's body, physically, emotionally, psychologically, or mentally.

Color therapy is distinct from other forms of light therapy, such as neonatal jaundice therapy and blood irradiation therapy, which are medically approved medical treatments for a variety of disorders, and from photobiology, the empirical study of the effects of light on living organisms.

Chromotherapy is a pseudoscience; practitioners believe that exposure to specific light colors will make people feel better physically or psychologically, but this has not been confirmed by scientific, peer-reviewed investigations.

So, it's easy to say that it's a color-based treatment, but how does it work? The color has been explored as a known medical treatment since 2000 B.C. It has always been known that colors affect patients' mood significantly, so much so that their clothes have been changed from white to blue or green, for example, by doctors. Its because white color induced nervousness among patients, whereas other colors provide quietness. But they affect not only the mood but also the thoughts and emotions. Colors can relax, encourage, excite, balance, or change our expectations, which has led them to be seen as therapeutic devices.

Methods of Delivery for Color Therapy

The alternative color therapy treatment technique focuses on transmitting the color light frequencies to the body. The light reaches the body either through the eyes or through devices for color therapy.

Through Eyes

One way to make the most of light therapy is to show the hue. Look at the color for a couple of minutes. That's all there is to delivery. Those colors you pick are what you need to be careful about. Green is considered the safest color. Red and orange will make you feel too anxious and agitated.

Color therapy is also individualized. What works to assist you could make someone else feel worse. If you have lots of anxiety and need to calm down, for example, blue might be an excellent color to use. However, if someone else were depressed, blue would not be a color that they should use in color therapy.

Via Color Therapy Equipment

There are different types of equipment for color therapy. Some of them can be quickly made, while others can be ordered for use by a color therapist. This appliance uses colored light projection. Often on a projector, the color is projected, and you are looking at it. The light comes from a specific 500-watt light bulb. The colored light can be shone on the skin with color therapy equipment, as well as modern and sometimes high-tech machinery that allows you to dial the color hue and intensity precisely.

Psychological Effects of Different Colors

Colors affect our mental processes, and our mood may change. Increasing intensity has a different effect, so for various mental disorders and mood issues, different colors are used. The following list describes how we are affected by the primary colors used in color therapy and what they can do for you.

Green

Green is the most equilibrated of all shades. Usually, color therapists consider green to be the safest color and usually start color therapy with it. Green will change your mood when you're feeling sad, helpless, or depressed. However, it is essential to have pure green color since a light green can tip into anxiety.

Green is said to enhance the feelings of love, happiness, and inner peace. It can bring hope, strength, and serenity to you. Green increases your wisdom and makes change and independence easier.

Blue

Blue is a color that needs to be used with particular caution because if you feel low, it can zap your strength. Blue does, however, help you to express your feelings, and is connected to your inner truth. Blue is a cold color that can help you feel more comfortable and calm. The blue is often used in meditation and relaxation therapy settings.

Blue can also be associated with spirituality, creativity, loyalty, and wisdom. A blue too dark or deep can lead to sadness, depression, and a sense of emptiness. It can also be used to aid in insomnia.

Yellow

Yellow can be used to bring strength in color therapy and to inspire action. You should feel better with this color. It can bring forth your understanding and wisdom. Yellows too bright or too vivid are synonymous with treason, cruelty, and paranoia. It can remind us that we are mortal. Yellow is the color with the most intensity in the spectrum.

Orange

Orange means plenty, enjoyment, health, and sexuality. Orange can be used to promote physical healing of different organs in the body. It gives you stamina and increased mental strength. It can increase your sense of bonding between your mind and body. Color therapists, however, usually avoid this color when one is prone to anxiety.

Red

Red is far more vivid than orange. It impacts emotional problems such as financial security and physical survival. It is mostly used for physical healing because it can have extreme psychological effects. Color therapists should not shine red on the head because it can cause extreme agitation. An expert color therapist can use infrared if done with caution. To anyone who has severe psychiatric disorders, neither red nor infrared is used.

Purple

Purple is tied to beauty, spirituality, and bliss. Violet is also used in color therapy on the forehead and neck to induce feelings of calm and relaxation. However, it is recommended for use on the body anywhere.

Chakra Healing with Crystals

The chakras are circular energy vortexes (or sometimes pictured as petalled flowers). They are your life force's focal points or prana – and their states are vital to your holistic well-being.

They affect nerves and major organs, as well as our emotional and spiritual condition. Ideally, all of our chakras should always be in balance, but that's rarely the case.

The Sanskrit word 'Chakra' translates literally to wheel or disc. In Yoga, Ayurveda, and meditation - The term refers to energy wheels all over the mind-body system. Imagine a swirling wheel of energy to visualize a Chakra in your body, which keeps you vibrant, healthy, and alive.

Consider this, why do we face challenges in so many aspects of our lives if we are all energetic beings of limitless potential? Why do our relationships, finances, career, and love life sometimes go awry?

The answer might be that the Chakra that controls this part of your life is dysfunctional, meaning it's your job to strengthen it.

Today, more and more people realize that Chakra Healing's ancient science holds the key to practically everything you've ever wanted in life. Have you ever wondered how certain people might use them?

Becoming a top performer at work almost effortlessly, have all the money they need for necessities and luxuries, and look fabulous while doing so? That's because they are secure in their 1st Chakra, which controls their career and finances.

Do you wonder how people indulge multiple times a week in mind-blowing lovemaking, even when they are swamped and married for years? Most likely, that their 2nd Chakra, which controls their sensuality and passion, is glowing.

Projecting an image of unwavering confidence consistently, even in the toughest situations, and play an active role in their families and communities? That is all thanks to their 3rd Chakra's radiance, which controls their power.

Do people enjoy energetic, caring, and understanding relationships with their teenage kids, partners, co-workers, friends, and settle any conflict in a friendly manner? Their 4th Chakra is undoubtedly healthy, controlling their relations.

Do they speak their minds always, wearing their hearts on their sleeves, and being respected for their authenticity? That's a shiny 5th Chakra at work, which controls the authentic voice.

Do they trust in their "good feelings" to solve problems intuitively at home, make critical decisions at work, and are correct at it most of the time? They have an efficient 6th Chakra that controls their intuition for that to thank.

Or those who experience an unwavering connection with God and their higher selves, and savor the security of knowing that they are watched over? Its 7th Chakra, which controls the divine consciousness, that is undoubtedly empowered.

The Chakras in Detail

Chakra root, Muladhara root, red.

The root chakra stands for our sense of security and safety.

Location: Spine Foundation

Influences primarily: Your career, mindset of money, and sense of belonging.

Energies: Earth, foundation, emphasis, centralization

Color: Red

Edges: Red and black gems like ruby, garnet, red jasper, and black tourmaline, bloodstone, and smoky quartz are very useful for balance. Of these crystals, ruby is the most powerful.

You know that when you enjoy your job, your Root Chakra is High, and you get praised for being so good at it. Everybody envies how you make, save, and invest money with your uncanny ability. You will have enough money to go on holiday and buy what you want without feeling guilty. Your friends and family always feel wanted and loved, and when you look in the mirror, you will feel good about yourself, both physically and emotionally.

If you know that when you're stuck in an unfulfilled and unrewarding career, your Root Chakra is WEAK or CLOSED, and you never seem to have enough money – which leaves you worried and in debt. Spending money is a frightening experience for you because you question your ability to make successful budgeting. You are suffering from weight or body problems that leave you in your skin, feeling unworthy and uncomfortable.

Chakra Sacra, Svadhisthana, Orange.

The sacral chakra stands for our creativity and our sexuality.

Location: Lower abdomen

Primarily Influences: The source of pleasure in water.

Energies: Heat, electricity, charging

Color: Orange

Gemstones: Orange gemstones such as carnelian, opal fire, and orange agate fit this Chakra well.

When you see closeness in a positive light as a high, pleasurable, and healthy activity, you know your Sacral Chakra is STRONG. With your partner, you share intense, regular, and lasting lovemaking. Orgasms are mind-blowing, and at the same time, you and your partner also orgasm. You make time at least a few times a week to be together, even if you've been attached to the same person for years. You will always attract the right partners – compatible people who feed you, fill you with joy, and make you a better person.

You know that your Sacred Chakra is Low or CLOSED when an intimate thought conjures feelings of remorse and pain in your mind. You may rarely have time or inclination to make love, and it's lackluster when you do. You and your partner never orgasm simultaneously, and premature or delayed ejaculation can be a common problem. You struggle to see yourself as magnetic, and also wonder if someone sees you that way. Sometimes, your partners are incorrect and incompatible for you, and you wonder if you will ever meet "the one."

The Chakra Solar Plexus, Manipura, The Yellow Colour.

The Solar chakra Plexus reflects our strength and self-esteem.

Location: On top of the navel.

Your power and channeling ability.

Energies: Fire, water, charging, energy efficiency.

Colour: Yellow.

Edges: Use yellow gems, such as amber, yellow or golden citrine, golden topaz, yellow sapphire, and lemon quartz for this chakra.

You know that your Power Chakra is STRONG when you are admired for your self-esteem and confidence, both in your career and in your personal life. You never fear to speak your mind, and you inspire those around you to do likewise. Your family, your colleagues, and your community see you as a charismatic individual, willing to use your energy and influence to make the world a better place.

Your Power in Chakra is WEAK or CLOSED while dealing with self-esteem problems and feelings of indignity. When confronted with critical decisions like moving to another city, changing your career, getting married to your partner, or having children, you tend to question yourself. You feel like one of the world's victims, and you often feel powerless about circumstances and the desires of others. You may also experience frequent stomach pains and worry about your stomach.

The heart chakra, Green, Anahata.

The chakra of Heart stands for love and acceptance.

Location: Chest center.

Primary Influences: Love, relationships, and acceptance of oneself.

Energies: Water, soothing, calming, relaxing.

Color: Green.

Edges: Use green, pink gems like rose quartz, green jade, emerald, peridot.

When you enjoy healthy, loving, and empathetic relationships at home, at work, and in your community, you know your Heart Chakra is STRONG! You and your family get along. Your friends consider you to be a reliable person. You're perceived at work as the one people are comfortable to talk to. You feel a sense of heartfelt gratitude for how beautiful your life is and feel compassion for everything around you.

You know that your Heart Chakra is WEAK or CLOSED the moment you tend to sabotage your affection with distrust, anger, and a sense that you will lose your independence if you rely too much on others. You may be struggling with commitment, experiencing frequent fights or misunderstandings with your loved ones, and always remaining "on guard" in case someone hurts you.

Chakra of the Throat, Vishuddha, Blue.

The Chakra of the Throat stands for honesty and contact.

Main Influences: The Chakra of the Throat controls the self-expression.

Place: The Throat.

Energies: Water, soothing, calming, relaxing.

Color: Light Blue.

Gemstones: Here are useful blue gemstones such as turquoise, blue apatite, and aquamarine.

"The Chakra of your "true voice."

You know that your Throat Chakra is STRONG when you are good at expressing your thoughts, ideas, and emotions. You are respected for your determination, excellent communication skills, and willingness to speak the truth, even though some may find it awkward. It enriches your career and your personal life.

You know that your Throat Chakra is WEAK or CLOSED when you always feel that no one cares about your opinions and that you have nothing worth saying. In your professional and social circles, you are likely to be known as the 'quiet one,' and you frequently settle for following others' opinions. Often you experience a blocked and sore throat.

Third Eye Chakra, Ajna, Indigo.

The Chakra of the Third Eye stands for creativity and intuition.

Primary Influences: This Chakra affects your intuition.

Location: Center of the forehead.

Energies: Air, meditative, intuitive, mindfulness.

Colour: Indigenous.

Gemstones: The most powerful are the indigo gemstones such as iolite and sapphire.

This Chakra acts as a compass within you.

You know that your Intuitive Chakra is STRONG when you can make precise, intuitive decisions and assessments about your career, your family, and other people's intentions. You always know things without knowing exactly how you know them, and in everything that you do, you have a clear sense of direction and consistency. You may have a vivid picture of where your life is going, and the people around you are likely to count on guidance and advice from you.

You know that your Intuitive Chakra is WEAK or CLOSED when faced with decisions and appeals for justice, you feel lost and helpless. You are indecisive, uncommitted, and unconfident about the choices that you end up making, as you have a history of making the wrong ones. You feel spiritually lost and unsure about your real purpose. You often get headaches in your brow region and deal with stress.

Indigo stimulates inner peace, depth, and devotion to the emotions.

Crown Chakra, Sahaswara, Violet or White.

The Crown chakra is an illumination, a spiritual connection, and a connection to our higher selves.

Primary Influences: This chakra influences your source connection.

Location: Top of the head.

Color: Violet or Clear.

Energies: Air, meditative, intuitive, mindfulness.

Gemstones: Use violet or white gemstones such as amethyst, clear quartz, and diamonds for this all-important chakra.

The Chakra of divine consciousness.

You know that your Crown Chakra is STRONG when you feel connected to a higher power perpetually, be it God, Universal Consciousness, or only your higher self. You are always reminded as you go about the daily life that you are being watched, and you feel immense gratitude for the ultimate love and appreciation you feel for yourself and others. Others call you "gluttonous."

You know that, when you feel little or no connection to a higher power, your Crown Chakra is WEAK or CLOSED, and you always feel alone. You feel unworthy of spiritual help and maybe even angry that your higher self might have abandoned you. You often experience migraines and headaches from tension.

Cleansing Crystals

Why do we need our crystals cleaned? There are two reasons; the first is to clean out the physical dirt and dust from our exciting new crystals. Often, new crystals have sand on them, from sitting in a store or market stall that needs removal. Secondly, we must also be vigorous in cleaning them. Why? You need to remove the energy left on the crystal from other people because many other people probably handled it before you bought the gem.

Here are eight ways to make your crystals clean:
1. Breath

When you buy your crystal first, one of the simplest methods of instant cleaning is holding your crystal in your hands, and then gently blow your breath on the crystal to clean it. You are adding your life-force energy onto the crystal as you do this, and this will remove and negate all the power left by other people; this will not remove physical dirt and dust.

2. Clean water

Can wash most of the crystal in running water. A word of caution, crystals can dissolve in water; some examples are selenite, kyanite, and azurite, or any of the soft crystals. You can use a damp cloth for these to wipe away the physical dirt. Some books will advise you to use seawater or spring water, but often that is not practical, so use the purest water you can, with little or no chemicals inside. It's recommended that you wash the physical dirt from all of your crystals regularly. It is often overlooked if you use the method of cleaning by sunlight or moonlight.

3. Sunlight

Place your crystals in the early morning sun to energize your crystals and cleanse them. A word of caution, when left in the sun too often for too long, gems like amethyst and fluorite will fade. It is also a good idea to use a piece of net to cover your crystals so the birds won't take them.

4. Moonlight

Place your crystal on a full moon outside to infuse moon energy into it. Moon force is soft feminine energy, so its cleansing is a very gentle way. It is a wonderful idea to cover them with a piece of net so the animals won't take them at night.

5. Earth Cleansing

Another standard method is burying your natural crystal. Some say that's the only way forward. With this method, there are a few precautions, remember where you are hiding them and do not bury them too deeply. Sometimes you may not find them again as Mother Earth reclaims them. The right way is to keep or conceal them is in a pot so that they can be found easily. When you dig them up, you'll need to rinse them off, as they'll have dirt on them.

6. Smudging

White sage has been in use for many years by native cultures for washing and is a compelling way to clean many crystals at once. If you have an extensive collection, putting them out into the moonlight would take you all night. They may be smudged with a white sage smudge stick or white sage incense. Light your stick of incense or smudge, and wave the smoke over your crystals. Sandalwood incense is a good cleanser, too. If you don't like these fragrances, your crystals can be washed with almost any incident. Even you can use resin on a block of charcoal, frankincense, myrrh, or a unique blend of crystal cleaning are good choices. You can close the room door when using resin and charcoal blocks and do the entire room at once.

7. Reiki

When you've been tuned to Reiki, you can use Reiki energy for crystal healing. If you are a level 1 Reiki, hold the crystals in your hands and send Reiki Healing to your gems with intention. Use your Reiki symbols over your crystals for level 2 practitioners, and then send them Reiki.

8. Other Crystals

The amethyst flat clusters are great for putting with other crystals; they will be energetically cleaned just by leaving your jewels on the amethyst for a few hours. Geodes and Transparent Quartz clusters are suitable for use as well.

It doesn't matter which tool you use, remember this is something to do and clean all your crystals regularly, both physically and energetically. Clean them always after healing or after using them on yourself.

The Power of Crystals

The awe of crystals are in the gems. I never got into collecting toys or dolls as a child; I had collected rocks! My collection of stones was quite impressive; I've had crystals and geodes from around the world. Not gathering your usual thing, but I don't think I was your average child either. I had been drawn to those gemstones for some reason. I was drawn to their sheer beauty, but I was drawn to something else about these enigmatic natural formations. I think those were the energies of those crystals that drew me to them. I started to read about the healing powers of crystals when I became an adult, and ultimately became a certified crystal healer.

Crystal therapy is using crystals to cure and bring about beneficial changes in mind, body, and spirit. For me, crystals cured sickness, healed emotional trauma, helped me overcome addictions, energized me, and completely changed my life! All gemstones hold their unique vibrational frequencies, and you can then alter your vibrational frequency by positioning them on your body or in your aura. Crystals serve as amplifiers too. They reinforce your purpose and deliver the desired result so much faster.

There are several different crystals of all shapes, sizes, and colors out there, and they each have their unique properties to resolve various physical and emotional issues. You can drive yourself mad, trying to explore and find the exact crystals you think you need. In reality, you can do it the other way around; the crystal picks you! So, if you're in a crystal shop picking up gems to take home with you, stop and go back to the first crystal you've encountered because it was definitely the crystal you've picked.

There are some preparations after you buy your new natural artifacts that need to be completed before they are ready for use. I'm sure you're probably excited and already want to use them, but these next steps are a crucial part of the process of crystal healing.

You will first need to clean your crystals of any negative energy it has absorbed. If they were in a store, they might have been touched by a lot of people, and the crystal could easily have absorbed any negative energies they were carrying, and you certainly don't want that in your energy field. Depending on how you use these, you will need to clean your crystals from time to time. Efficient methods for removing crystals are numerous. The easiest and most effective way is to place them in your hands, holding the intention of clearing all the negative energy from the crystal and keeping it for one to two minutes under running water. The faucet works just fine. Some other cleaning methods include placing them in salt for several hours, or burying them in the earth for a day or two, or only using your breath.

Step two is to attune the new crystal to your vibrational frequency and set the intention that it will be used only for your higher good or for the right of anyone else who uses it. All you need to do is put your hands together on the crystal, close your eyes, and set those two intentions. You can either say it aloud or think about it; either way is successful.

Step three involves charging your crystals. Put the crystals in direct sunlight for at least 5 hours. You can also put them under the brightness of a full or new moon, overnight.

The final step is to program the crystals to what you'll use them for. For example, you can say they are to be used for general healing or protection purposes, or grounding, etc. It may or may not be an optional step. The reason one can do this step is because programming a crystal for a specific use further changes it to the frequency of your needs, bringing about the desired result even faster. To do this, you must keep the crystal in your hands and say, "This crystal will be used for... (say your intentions here)," aloud (not in your head), and fill in the blank. To program the crystal in full, repeat those words 3 to 4 times. You're now ready to use your new crystals!

There are many ways you can use your crystals; it all depends on your needs. Here are few ways you can use your precious gemstones: you can wear them as a necklace or bring one or two of them with you in your pocket or purse (if you use them this way, note that you need to clean your crystals more frequently as they can soak up any negativity in the world in which you are). You can also meditate with your crystals by putting them on or around you, and your meditation will be significantly intensified. By placing corresponding stones on each chakra and intending to clear and balance them, you can adjust and clear your chakras using crystals. For clearing or security, you can hold crystals around your room or in your workspace. You can even put some stones under your pillow at night to enhance and recall your dreams, or to sleep better. The possibilities with crystals are endless, and they will surely improve your life in every field! I hope you like to use the crystals just as much as I do!

Crystal Gridding

Another way to gain the healing powers of crystals is by using them in a grid formation. It is supposed to make the power and energy of each used crystal stronger and more powerful, so it's a great way to clear up a whole room in your home.

Crystal Grids are a beautiful and incredibly powerful way to manifest your dreams, goals, and intentions. A crystal grid's strength comes from the combined energies of the crystals you're using, how you lay them out, and the goals you set. A crystal grid is a proper understanding of crystals and stones used to manifest the desired result. Keep in mind that the world wants to give us what we need and not just what we want. So, it is best to focus on manifesting a need vs. a want if you would like it to come to fruition. People use collective intentions for well-being, abundance, healing, and protection for crystal grids.

When it comes to crystal grids, there are no hard and fast rules; it's best to use your work and intuition with what you feel directed to do with the crystals. Some people like to do them with sacred geometry on a cloth or piece of paper, as they genuinely think this increases the grid's power. Some prefer to incorporate bits of nature into their systems, such as leaves or flowers. Many people pick their stones based on the individual crystal properties that align with what they'd like to manifest. The choices are limitless! Below is the commonly used technique for a crystal grid, which may be beneficial for beginners. The grid patterns are geometric, and online models can be found for them. Do not get this confused with any witchcraft or hocus pocus magic. It is an excellent means of harnessing the crystals' full energy. The crystals 'communicate' with each other, and replace with positive energy all negative energy in the room. It would be best if you contemplated what your intention is to make the grid before creating your grid. While creating your grid, you can either state your intent loudly or, likewise, write it down on a piece of paper, so you're focused. The intention could be anything you wish for or dream of, such as health, affection, fertility, clarity, focus, etc.

What Crystals To Use

The first crystal to choose from is the center stone, which is often called the master crystal. That crystal is the one that communicates in the grid to the other gems. It needs a lot of energy to hold, and some people prefer to use pyramid or cluster crystals for this position.

The next crystal to select is what is called the 'activation wand'. It is the crystal on which you focus your aim. Being the same type of crystal as one of the other in the grid is helpful for this crystal. You can write their name on a piece of paper and place it on the grid below the master crystal if you want to do long-distance healing, either for a person or a place (or maybe a country that has suffered a tragic disaster).

The remainder of the crystals you want to use will depend on the purpose that you concentrate on. For example, if romance and love are your goals, use the crystals that suit those emotions and thoughts. Alternatively, you can use a pendulum to help you pick the correct gems, or listen to your instincts and choose the ones you think you should choose. Some people tend to put transparent quartz crystals to amplify the energy on the grid's outer points.

Position Your Grid

You want to place your grid in an area that is not going to be disrupted. It may be a quiet corner of a house, or if you have an altar of meditation or a holy place in your home, these are the right places for your grid. Some think putting the grid in the room's northern region makes the energy stronger, but that's not important.

Activating Your Grid

It's time to activate the grid once your system is set up with the crystals you have selected. A step-by-step guideline on the ways to practice is here:

1. For 5 minutes, meditate or relax, so that you can ground yourself.
2. Take hold of the wand and then state your intent or positive reinforcement, concentrating heavily on what you want to be the product.
3. Now take a moment to accept that your purpose, called 'programming,' is real.
4. Wait a few minutes, then put your wand down, and activate the grid.

Next, take time to sit in front of your grid each week and relax or even better, meditate, and focus on your original intention. You can leave your grid the same way for weeks, but if you feel it is losing its strength, you can recharge it. To restore the crystals and their energy, perform a new activation. When you feel like the grid has done what you wanted it to do, and the goal becomes concrete, remember to say thanks to the grid and crystals. You may continue the cycle with a new goal once again when you feel it is time.

Think using crystal therapy for the daily grind survival

At times life can be quite stressful. Going to the office every-day and taking care of other responsibilities can virtually drain your energy. You may feel frustrated with daily disappointments ranging from illness, professional issues, and issues of love, and even from the pressures of a written examination or promotion. If you want to take a healing break from these things, then crystal therapy may be used. You can use it to help you cure illness, balance energies, shield yourself from harmful energies, and even find love in this universe. Here are some essential points about crystal therapy, which you should know about.

The Basics of Crystal Therapy

The belief in crystal therapy is based on the idea that the balance of energies within us depends on individual crystals and charm stones. Of course, it's all based on the premise that we all have a kind of vibration energy system, and the use of these beautiful stones and crystals can be very useful in tuning this mechanism. In other words, these precious stones hold healing or magical forces inside them, and we can all use them on our own or with the aid of a crystal therapist. The efficiency of such therapy would be based not only on the ability to draw out the powers of a crystal but also on the chemical composition of the stone, its type, its color, its atomic structure, and its over physical form. It also means that a particular crystal may have special powers and can react to individual needs. However, there's the concept that a single charm stone typically contains not only one form of healing power, but many.

If you choose to use crystal therapy for a variety of therapeutic purposes, then here is a quick guide to different crystals and charm stones and their strengths.

1. Chakra Equalizers

There are individual crystals that can help in your energy balance. It is a good starting point if you don't already know which area of emphasis you'd like. You can then make use of jade, serpentine, and fulgurite as your chakra balancing stones to have a healthy disposition overall.

2. Love Crystals

If you want to support in the field of love, then you can use the crystals of love. The rose quartz, apatite, and cobalt calcite are the most popular. These charming stones give off warm and soft energies, so they are best for either attracting love or even helping those around you to be more caring.

3. Energizing Charm Stones

If you are a bit low in strength, then as part of your crystal therapy, you can use amulets, rings, or any other jewelry piece with opal or topaz stones. These stones of beauty will support you when you're tired and exhausted. Just be sure to keep them from your bedside so that you can relax for a good night.

4. Memory Keepers

Some stones help the memory retain a lot of information and so they are also called keepers of crystal record. Some examples include carnelians, garnets, and rubies. They can be quite useful when preparing for examinations.

5. Protective and Shielding Crystals

Diamonds, yellow jasper, and fluorite are the minerals with the highest defensive quality. They work best when worn as ornamental jewelry or when kept in the purse or pockets. These crystals work primarily by absorbing the negative energies around you, so it is also essential to know how to clean them from time to time.

The use of the crystals mentioned above is all part of crystal therapy that mainly aims at balancing the energy inside you. Crystal therapy is also known for soothing and calming the body and mind and improving the body's immune system.

Step-by-step Guide to Crystal Grid Creation

The first step is to choose what your grid is intended for. You might wish to write that down on a piece of paper and put it in your grid under the central stone. Try to be specific, what you will like, and try to stick with a need, as mentioned before, rather than want if you can.

Pick the crystals you want. You can do this while keeping in mind the individual properties of crystals and what your intentions are, but you can also work with anything you have on hand. Most importantly, trust your intuition and what you feel to use for guidance.

It's necessary to cleanse your crystals and the space you will be doing your crystal grid in. I enjoy doing this by using a sage smudge stick. However, there are different ways you can cleanse your crystals; you could use sound, like Tibetan singing bowls. Moonlight is another option. You can place the jewels in the light to wash them during the full moon. Others include burying your crystals in the earth, water, putting them in sunlight, using Reiki, or salt. Just be careful, some gems do not like water, like Selenite. Therefore, I prefer to stick to the sage.

Place the piece of paper you wrote down your intentions in the center of your space and say what your plans are whilst you do this, either in your mind or aloud. Take a moment and slow down while you are doing this, and connect with your spirit and the universal energy. You might wish to light a candle or play some relaxing music whilst doing this.

Some people feel it's best to start and go in from the outside, while others tend to start in the middle and work their way out. Start placing your crystals down and do whatever feels right for you. Some people like using sacred geometry to do this, and it gives them an easy guide on where their crystals can be placed.

The last step is to switch on your grid. I like to do this with a clear quartz base. It is sort of like a dot-to-dot energetic, as you touch each gem with your point, drawing an invisible line to join them to each other. It is safer to keep your crystal grid in place for some time, instead of moving it straight away. I prefer to leave mine for at least 48 hours but do something that works for you. Some people would give them up in the long run. They are sure to make an excellent addition to any space.

How long am I going to keep the grid?

The better, the longer! The best thing about crystal grids is its long service life. It would help if you considered making your crystal grids a part of home decoration. They're beautiful, realistic, and helpful. If they are permanent, grids that encourage abundance, health, and security are most active. Your crystal grids need not be stable to produce unbelievable results, however.

For instance, if you're putting together a crystal grid for a particular event, there's no reason it's permanent. A good thumb rule is to assemble the grid about a day before and take it down about a day after it's finished. As a form of meditation, you could even make a crystal grid, and disassemble it when you're done.

How big do crystal grids need to be?

Again, this is a highly personal and situational thing. When using sacred geometry, a minimum of three "layers" of crystals is the best practice. You could make crystal grids that are as large as people, depending on the size of the space! Or just as little as a coaster. Note the essential aspect of this is the purpose behind creating a crystal grid. I saw crystal grids as big as dinner plates, whole backyards, and everything in between. In crystal grids and sacred geometry bigger doesn't automatically equal better. It is not precisely the Universe that needs a massive grid to understand what your intent is. So, go for whatever size you feel like suits you best.

Should I use crystals that are tumbled, rough, or pointed?

Why not all 3? Tumbled stones usually give off more subtle and gentle energies. Rough stones tend to be bigger, so they seem to have a "stronger" energetic force. It is believed that pointy crystals direct their energy in a specific direction, wherever the ending goes. These are the masses' standard views.

I love to include all types of crystals in my grids. Some gems don't come in a tumbled form, and they can be hard to find. You may find that for specific intentions, rough stones work better over others. And pointed crystals can help to overcharge the energy of the other rocks in the grid. Thus, all three have a place in grid production.

Crystals to Help You Sleep

If you notice that you have trouble getting to sleep, then we may have the solution: crystals for you. Perhaps you never thought of using them as a solution, but you'd be shocked at how they might help. So, if you find yourself turning and twisting through the night, then start reading for a natural way to sleep. The most potent gams to help you sleep are the Amethyst, sodalite, Jade, Clear Quartz, and selenite. So, let's see how you can profit from each of these.

Amethyst

Amethyst is a crystal that brings both soothing and calming energies to help you sleep. It works by consuming and repelling all harmful energies that could disturb your sleep. It enables you to relax by repelling those dangerous sources and removing your body from stress and anxiety. It can also help soothe stress and nervous energies and help you sleep. You can also increase your dreams by placing Amethyst under your pillow before you go to sleep, which enables you to remember your dreams and chases away any nightmares that might keep you up.

Sodalite

Sodalite provides a sense of order and calmness. Sodalite can help avoid insomnia, too.

Clear Quartz

Clear Quartz can help make sure you have pleasant dreams while you sleep. It is because it is a gemstone that stimulates and energizes by magnifying the properties of all other crystals that strike it. Which means it will amplify Selenite and Amethyst's soothing powers in crystal bags. This crystal can help you concentrate on your dreams too. Before you sleep, you can keep your quartz crystal in your pocket, and consider any questions or issues that you might have. Then, when you fall asleep, the crystals beneath the pillow can ease your mind while you sleep and work through these problems.

Smokey Quartz-Dispels the hallucinations and lets the dreams manifest. It disperses terror, raises depression and negativity. It also brings emotional calm, and soothes stress and anxiety.

Selenite

Furthermore, it is believed that selenite is one of the best crystals to help with insomnia. This crystal works by filling your body with calming energy when you sleep, rejuvenating, and cleaning your aura, so you feel refreshed and well-rested when you wake up. The selenite in the crystal bag will work to continually reactivate and cleanse the crystals that contact it, which will keep them free of harmful energy.

Jade

A "dream stone," Jade makes insightful dreams come true. It helps the release of emotions, particularly irritability.

Crystal system for sleeping well

Why not try crystals first, before you reach for over-the-counter medicines to help you sleep? Seeking natural ways to help you relax, rather than medication, as they are much more useful for your body. It is because you'll be able to reprogram your body and mind and create better long-term sleep patterns.

It's essential to get rid of any built-up frustrations you have because of sleeping difficulty before you sleep. Silently sit down and keep your crystals in your hands for a couple of minutes and take a deep breath, imagine yourself and your crystals surrounded by white light and feel the crystals' soothing force. Set your jewels in mind; let them know precisely what you need them to help you with. You may even like to have it written down. Also, making sure you clean your crystals if they're new, and every now and then while using them, is essential.

Pleasant collection for Sweet dreams

If you want to try crystals to help make your sleep better, then why not browse our selection today. After a good night's sleep, we have a wide range of beautiful crystals that can help you feel refreshed and awaken. Our beautiful Sweet Dreams Set is perfect for keeping under your pillow or beside your bed while you sleep. Or you may choose one of our powerful crystal grids. Even if you only have one of the crystals mentioned above, it can help you get better nights of sleep.

Crystal Grid for Your Home

Crystal Grids are a considerable way to set your intentions, manifest your goals, promote healing, or impact a space's energy. But did you know your house can be bridged? It is a perfect way to build a healthy atmosphere and prevent harmful energy from harming yourself and your home. And we sell beautiful Home Gridding Sets that include everything you need to make things super easy.

Here's our simple step-by-step gridding guide for your home;
Step one:

Give the right clean to your home. Where possible, remove any dust, rubbish, or clutter. Smudge every room within the house once your house is clean. The White Sage Smudge Stick in your Home Gridding Package will do this. Start the back of the house and wave the smoke in the corners of the room and up to the ceiling. As you go, see negative and unwanted energies drifting out of your space with wild smoke. Focus on your intentions; let the sage guide you as you smudge from room to room to the entrance of your home.

Step two:

Place your crystals with intentions. Hold your crystals in hand, and clear any negativity from your mind. You may want to do a breathing exercise, or meditate for a few minutes with your crystal. Choose an intention that is good for your short and long-term goals, trying to be neither too specific nor too materialistic. A rule of thumb is to focus on your need, then ask the Universe anything. You can set the intention, for example, that your crystals help protect your home from any negative people or energies—focus on your crystal with a still mind and purpose. You might want to describe your intention aloud or repeat it in your head, focusing consistently on the link between your words and your crystal. Or you might opt to write down your plans on a piece of paper. Some people are even fond of keeping their crystals above their Third Eye as they set their purpose. Again, it would help if you did what you feel is right. Continue until your mind and body feel set to your goal.

Step three:

You can now start putting the crystals around your house. Start by putting in the four corners of your home one Black Tourmaline Tumble, one White Quartz Tumble, and one Selenite Tumble. If your home isn't a perfect square, you can also place the stones in the north, south, east, and west. Those crystals will help to absorb any negative energy. Selenite will help cleanse the other minerals.

Step four:

Place your twin Red Tiger Eye Tumbles in front of you. Ideally, it should be visible just inside. The Red Tiger Eye protects against the evil eye and attacks at home or while on a journey. So, when you travel, you can even take these with you, if you like. It's also the charm of money!

Step five:

Next, you will create the outside of the grid by placing the remaining Selenite Tumbles in between each Black Tourmaline, on the border of your house, or the windowsill. Think of it as you build a square pattern all-around your home. The corners are Black Tourmaline, Clear Quartz, and Selenite, and more Selenite Tumbles make up the sides.

If you've got a large house, you may want to buy two of the Home Gridding Packages. If you have walls in your way, just use discretion/intuition about where the stones are best positioned. Trusting in one's gut feelings is always best. After all, it is your home. Now your home grid is set, some people like placing a crystal in their home's center, and then it's energy and properties can be amplified throughout the house. Depending on your mood and what you might be attempting to manifest at the moment, this crystal will change. It is just like the center stone's energy is amplified, and the focus is making any crystal grid.

While selenite does not need charging in your grid and will help keep the other stones clean, it is always a great idea to clean your crystals at least once a month.

The Crystal Power

Crystals have always been seen as a source of strength — and as a gift from the gods. Whatever their size, impressive gems hold an aura of mystery and authority. Gemstones have symbolized wealth from prehistory to the present, and have granted remarkable properties. The ancient texts which tell us so much about the power of stones originated in the Stone Age, a time when technology came from rocks quite literally. We've continued to harness their magical power ever since. In the year 1714, M. B. Valentini's Museum imagined an airship built in 5(five) years by a Brazilian priest; the craft was to be propelled by agate and iron, which would become magnetic when heated up in the sun. Our present technology does not exist without crystals as odd as this might seem; they power computers and surgical instruments, coat engines, and spaceships. Crystals are the foundational building blocks of science and art. The ancients attributed healing ability to crystals. Those remedies were passed on by the Greek philosopher Theophrastus and the Roman geographer Pliny (though Pliny denounced some as false claims). The Babylonians attributed the fate of humanity to the influence of precious stones. Our ancestors claimed that the Earth covered by spheres of crystal in which gods, stars, and planets dwelt. The color or constitution of a crystal, or its planetary affiliation, initially indicated its effectiveness for specific conditions. Unfortunately, difficulties in translation often make it impossible to determine precisely which stone early texts mentioned, but some references are crystal clear.

Each crystal has a unique signature in terms of energy. Those "light templates" are encoded with everything you need to activate your power. The aim is to find a crystal that fits your energy or elevates your spiritual resonance to ensure the health and enhance your consciousness.

The Power of Gems

Flashy gemstones not only carry strength. Crystals of all kinds have served as protective amulets since antiquity. Humble stones like Flint were magical carriers for the soul, for metaphysical operations, or the use of shamans on their journeys throughout the world. Many stones produced or could be superheated by incandescent sparks into streams of gold, silver, copper, and other precious metals. The sky rocks that fell to Earth were just as beautiful, taking iron with them to forge instruments and build weapons. Egyptologist Wallis Budge explained, "Each stone had a kind of living personality that will experience sickness, disease, and will become old and powerless, and even die." But stones could also heal in Egyptian medicine. The Greek philosopher Plato believed that rocks were living beings produced by the process of fermentation induced by "a life-giving intelligence coming down from the stars." According to myths, crystals solidified from ice, a view strengthened by water bubbles sometimes found within a crystal.

The Power of Magic

Crystals were also credited with having magical strength, as seen in the quotation above from a stone book from the third century B.C.E. It also describes the awe and reverence with which they were treated. Magic is not merely superstition — it is the foundation for the experimental sciences highly valued by the modern world. We wouldn't have medicine, astronomy, literature and drama, chemistry, mathematics, music, mythology, and perhaps even religion itself without magic. Magical formulae are some of the oldest writings, and it could be argued that the alphabet — even knowledge recording itself — is a form of magic. Magic is not just a set of beliefs and practices; it is a way of looking at the world. Ancient life and death were governed by the view that the natural world was animate, alive with magic forces interpenetrating the substance of the physical and the metaphysical realms. Today the crystal workers still interact within crystals with animate troops, the living beings. The word magic comes from magi, Persia, and Babylon's wise men and women, but it's rooted in the Sumerian world image meaning "deep." Magic was a way to manipulate the everyday world and attracting the favor of the gods, but also, as the anthropologist Robert Ranulph Marett tells us, "a higher level of experience." In which spiritual enlargement is valued for its own sake. "This book deals with this spiritual expansion (the cycle of growth), as well as with the therapeutic and transformative properties of crystals.

CHAPTER SIX

Ways To Spot Real Crystal From Glass

C rystal awards will bring an additional touch of prestige to the ceremony while trying to honor employee achievements or an exceptional accomplishment on the football field. When comparing crystal awards, make sure that the prize is crystal and not glass or synthetic material, like Lucite. Whether you have a glass or a crystal award is easy to tell.

There are about five significant differences between crystal awards and glass awards made from the material of lesser quality. Crystal has thick metals, and it's going to be thicker than glass or lucite. Compare crystal with a glass which is similar in size-the the crystal should be significantly more substantial.

Another way of knowing whether it is glass or the real thing is to check its resonance. Tap a piece of crystal, and a high-pitched tone will emit while a glass or Lucite plaque will sound like a low-pitched kludge. The tone of the crystal piece should be of a slight timbre.

Crystal and glass refract light differently, as well. Hold a crystal up to the sun, and it should look reasonably clear, but when held at certain angles to the light, it should also show a rainbow prism. Glass can also have a prism effect because when the sun goes through, the transparent glass may have a slightly green or yellow tint.

Look closely at the sides and angles of a plaque with crystals. A crystal will have smooth, rounded edges and cuts while the edges and corners of a glass piece will be sharp-angled. It is because the glass is much simpler to work with, and is less costly, so breakage and flaws in the production process are more appropriate. Crystal fabrics are much more valuable.

Again, as glass is easier to work with than crystal when compared with the glass version, the crystal award tends to be thicker and sturdier. If the prize feels weak and flimsy, it is most likely glass or anything other than the crystal. If it feels a bit thicker and more substantial, then it is most likely the real thing .

When deciding whether a prize is made from crystal or glass, it is necessary to note that the above rules are just guidelines, verify that all are checked when comparing shopping. At first glance, glass and crystal are hard to tell but keep these rules in mind, and it will be almost impossible to mistake glass for a crystal.

What Is Crystal Lead-Free?

When people think of high-end crystal, they think of traditional leaded crystal — for example, a wine glass with that beautiful, somewhat heavy feel that sparkles with faceted brilliance, and the beautiful, sing-songy ring that resonates when you tap it. It was an only leaded crystal that produced these exquisite attributes for a very long time. While lead crystal is still trendy, there is another type of high-quality glass that can offer the same experience.

Normal Glass

Which is known as soda-lime glass is "natural" glass such as traditional water glass, beer glass, glass baking dish, etc. Not exceptionally brilliant or beautiful, but functional, and much longer-lasting than crystal in most cases. Soda-lime Glass consists of several main ingredients — sodium carbonate, lime, dolomite, silicon dioxide, and aluminum oxide, and smaller amounts of other parts called "fining agents," which are melted together in a furnace at a very high temperature. The melted liquid sits down to allow the bubbles in it to rise out of it — this is called "fining out." The glass is then formed using various processes depending on the final product's purpose, i.e., drinking glass, window panel, windshield, etc. Lead is added to traditional crystal.

Crystal Lead

Traditional lead crystal glass adds to the usual glass mix — lead oxide, another ingredient. Using lead creates a few select properties that make the glass "crystal." Soda glass contains non-structural molecules — which is known as amorphous. There's no particular order, but it's closely connected, making soda-lime glass more resilient. The lead-crystal particles have a distinct three-dimensional structure. These molecules create the brilliance of the sparkling bottle. The crystal has a higher "refractive index" than standard glass, and making the index brilliant. Adding lead to the glass often helps it melt at a lower temperature, which allows it to consume less energy than soda. It is why when you tap the crystal, it rings.

Free Crystal Lead

Although it will possibly still be used by lead crystal purists, there is now an alternative with the same characteristics. It offers a choice for those who enjoy high-quality crystal but worry about lead content in everything that contains consumables. It is especially applicable in decanters, which I will follow up in a little bit. The lead is replaced with barium oxide (BaCO3) when making lead free crystal glass. The introduction of barium oxide creates a glass with a comparatively high refractive index, increasing its brilliance. Often, barium oxide is lighter than lead oxide, rendering the glass thinner with nearly equal longevity. As mentioned before, for those concerned about the content of lead in their crystal glassware, such only raises a health question for crystal decanters. The reason for this is that wine and spirit guides are typically kept longer in decanters than a glass of wine. It creates a more significant time window for lead to leach from it, possibly. For a long time, I haven't stored wine in the decanters — it's more about aeration and demonstration for me — so I'm not concerned about the issue.

Crystal Lead vs. Free Crystal Lead

Whether you want to pick one over the other is always just a matter of personal preference. There are many manufacturers of high-end crystals who make exquisite glass free from lead. I have used the weight variance frequently, and the only significant difference that I have found is: In a good quality crystal bottle, wines taste much better than a standard drinking glass every day of the week.

Bohemian and Crystal Waterford

Crystal giftware has been the epitome of the gift-giving and showing appreciation to a friend or loved one since its inception centuries ago.

Combining a beautiful crystal set with a bottle of wine or champagne is a practical and easy gift solution that has been able to withstand the test of time. Simplicity's brilliance has allowed crystal gifts to stand the test of time and remain as popular as ever. Bohemian Crystal and Waterford Crystal have become synonymous with crystal giftware, and have established themselves as tradition honored by both leaders of this time.

Bohemian Crystal production began in Czechoslovakia (formerly known as Bohemia) due to the abundance of natural resources in the countryside. Potash discovered by Bohemian glass cutters combined with chalk produced a transparent colorless glass that was more durable than Italian glass. It was at this time that, for the first time in history, the term Bohemian crystal arose to differentiate its qualities from glass coming from other countries. One could cut this unique Czech glass with a wheel.

Bohemia became the breeding ground for skilled artisans who worked artfully with crystal. Bohemian crystal became famous for its superb cutting and gravure. They became expert glass-making teachers in neighboring and remote countries. A technical glass-making school system was created by the middle of the 19th century, which encouraged traditional and innovative techniques like professional preparation.

Bohemia looked at the export trade and mass-produced colored glass for shipment worldwide in the second half of the 19th century. Vase pairs were either produced in a single opaque glass color or two-colored cased glass. These have been decorated in thickly enameling flower subjects that are painted at high speed. Others have been decorated with colorful lithographic prints that copy famous paintings. Such glass items were manufactured in massive quantities in large factories and were available in all of Europe and America by mail order. They were not considered fine art but also provided cheap decorative objects for brightening up ordinary homes; reverse glass painting was a Czech specialty. Here the image is carefully hand-painted on the back of a glass panel using a variety of techniques and materials to mount the picture in a beveled wooden frame. Glass craftsmanship remained high even under the Communists because it was not considered an ideological threat to communism.

This continued excellence standard has enabled the products to maintain their reputation for centuries as a premium in gift ideas. With Bohemian glassware's unique characteristics combined with centuries of glass cutting experience, each piece has a reputation for making a lasting impression. A present's real value is how highly regarded as the receiver maintains his gift after time. Bohemian Crystal almost always finds its way to the centerpiece of any display cabinet and creates a lasting impression even when not in use.

Czechoslovakia has produced many experts in the cutting of beautiful glass. Few will be as influential as Charles Bacik on the art. Amid this tradition, Charles grow up and learn the secrets of fantastic glass cutting and crystal ware to open numerous factories specializing in it. However, as the Communists had taken over his factories after WW2, he immigrated to Ireland. In 1947 he started Waterford Glass in partnership with a Dublin gift-shop owner, Bernard Fitzpatrick. The firm was in financial difficulties in 1950, and ceded ownership to the Irish Glass Bottle Company. He kept working as a consultant for the company until 1974, and as a member of the board until 1984. Under his leadership and direction, Crystal Waterford would become one of the undisputed leaders in the making of crystal gifts.

Waterford Crystal currently designs, manufactures and markets a wide variety of crystal stemware, barware, and giftware for sale worldwide. In recent years, by expanding into several new businesses, Waterford has built on its reputation as a leading supplier of prestigious tabletop and gift produce. With the launch of the Marquis by Waterford, significant expansions into tabletops and gifts took place. This initiative reflects the company's commitment to creating prestigious products, the classic designs that transcend time.

Today, Waterford Crystal has very close ties to its legendary predecessor. There is the same dedication to the purity of color, the same inspiration for the design, and the same pursuit of the highest possible quality levels. The traditional cutting patterns made famous by the Waterford artisans became the basis of design for the company's growing product range.

Today, Waterford Crystal is one of the leaders in premium crystal and creates elegant handmade crystal stemware, giftware, and lighting, designed and produced to the highest standards. People who are fortunate enough to have experienced Waterford Crystal find it the best for buying for themselves and as gifts.

It is impossible to choose between Bohemia or Waterford Crystal. Both companies have built a reputation based on products that are the result of centuries of craftsmanship and adaptation to new technology and methods to ensure that the customer receives the best available glassware. The customer can't go wrong, either when picking either.

How to Spot a Crystal with High-quality?

When it comes to glassware, people think that listening to the "ting" from the item is the best way to spot price. But if you educate your eyes to find a piece of high-quality quartz, you can give your ears the day off.

Why? For what? The sound of a "ting" from a piece of glass is subjective, and the quality of that piece of stemware may not be told, but to assess if you have the real thing, other considerations need to be evident.

Glassware (traditional soda-lime glass) contains approximately 50 percent silica (sand) without lead. Crystal includes a point of at least 24 percent. That is the fundamental distinction between glass and crystal.

Sounds pretty straightforward, but it's not, to be honest. You'll recall hearing your mother that nothing worth getting is ever easy.

Your daily orange juice glass is mostly made of a material called a soda-lime, a mixture of lime, silica (sand), and sodium. It's used for products like windows and daily drinking glasses. Most glasses made today in the United States are soda-lime glass and do not require a significant investment.

On the other hand, borosilicate glass-called Fire-glass in the early 1900s and now called Pyrex by its brand name-is a heat-resistant glass that does not break when exposed to extreme changes in temperature. It is costlier than soda-lime glass and was first used for freight train windshields to avoid breakage of windows when trains encountered radical weather changes.

Borosilicate glass is used primarily in laboratories and does not destroy quickly. Neither of these glass types - soda-lime glass or borosilicate glass - is considered crystal because there is no content of 24 percent lead.

Crystal consists of silica (sand), lead oxide, soda and is known to be beautiful and durable. "Crystal" is used to describe any glassware that looks fancy or used in champagne, wine, or spirits service. It is a choice for spirits and wine connoisseurs because it allows the drinker to evaluate the wine or liquor color and viscosity. If your piece of crystal is visible, it will possibly have a higher content of lead.

When it comes to crystal, the most important characteristics are its reflective nature and the 24 percent lead content. Crystal is more transparent than a typical piece of soda-lime glass, its reflective quality is why crystal is used for chandeliers, elegant wine glasses, and pendants for jewelry. Like those pieces made by high-quality companies like Waterford, the stunning gem may even exceed the requirement of 24 percent lead content. Those firms can supply products that are 30 percent or more in lead content.

The confusion surrounding crystal is historical and chemical-based. First of all, the crystal does not have a crystalline structure despite its name. Crystal is from the term "Cristallo" coined by Italian glassmakers at the famous Murano glass blowing center near Venice to define quality glassware that did not meet the European lead content standard.

Crystal is typically thin because glass with a high level of lead is more natural to sculpt. Point lowers the glass's working temperature, extending the time a glassblower has to carve one piece.

Tips to tell the gap between regular soda-lime glass and crystal:

- Crystal has the following characteristics: 24 percent lead content, bright reflective quality, silver or silver/purple hue, rainbow prism effect when kept to the view, thinner than regular soda-lime glass, and more substantial than regular soda-lime glass.

- Crystal will sparkle with a lead content of over 35 percent.

- Place your thumb in the piece's cut design, and if you move your thumb and cut it, you'll have a bit of crystal cut. Crystal should have sharp cutting properties.

- Beautiful glassware contains some lead content, but if the lead content level of 24 percent is reached, the manufacturer cannot, by law, call that piece "crystal."

Here Are Few Ways to Choose a Crystal That Is Right for You

You will find that the right crystal will call you out based on what you need, and this is always the best way to select a diamond.

We suggest you go to our Tumbled Stones page to follow this method, where you can see an extensive collection of stones at once. Then, follow the following steps:

1) Take note of any gems which instantly pop up at you. Please do not click on them and read nothing about them-simply write down their names. Here are some questions that will support you in this move.

Which one are you drawn to for its beauty?

When you move your eyes over all the different stones, which one tugs you energetically?

Which one feels like they are calling you out?

Which ones call to you to touch them?

2) Now spend some time looking at every particular stone (again without reading anything about it). Be on the lookout for these few things, as you do:

Note any emotions that come up when you look at a stone.

How does its look make you feel?

1) Please close your eyes and imagine holding it in your hand-notice whether your hand gets warm or you feel any sensations or subtle vibrations.
2) Ask for instruction from your higher self and follow your intuition.
3) Notice if any of those you immediately draw to make a lasting impression on you after looking at the picture. If so, then those are the ones to begin.
4) Click the stones you've been most drawn to in steps 1 and 2, Our guess is, you're going to be shocked how well they fit with what you're looking for right now in your life.

Crystals found inside stones or rocks;

Many rocks have or are known to have crystals found on their surfaces, inside the stones. Crystals have flat surfaces that can be small or large. It is said that crystals with small flat surfaces have "facets." All glasses have face surfaces, but not all crystals have multiple facets. There have been several excellent books and blogs published to help classify crystals on or inside the rocks. Collect numerous samples of rock with crystals before identification.

Wash the rocks gathering with water. Use an old toothbrush to remove any dirt within the stone's fissures or cracks.

Wipe the rocks with a soft cloth. Let the stones sit, until dry, for 30 minutes.

Using a magnifying lens, look at the crystals in the rock.

Use a book to classify the types of minerals and crystals in the minerals you are studying.

Scrutinize the crystals of the rock, and compare them with the pictures in the book. Find the one in your rock which looks most like the crystal.

I am using the same method of using the Internet to classify the rocks and crystals. Search also for websites for the identification of stone, crystal, or rock and crystal. Use a magnifying lens to display the glass. Compare it to internet photos of crystals.

Take the rock, already washed, to the local school system. Ask to speak with the science teacher at the high school. Show the stone to the science teacher, and ask for their opinion. Look at any books that the science teacher may have about the association with the rock.

3. Jade Cove, California

Unlike the first two locations on this list, Jade Cove — located in California's Big Sur area — is not sold out. On the contrary, there are barriers to entry here: the way down is steep and potentially dangerous; sometimes, signs for pointing the way are missing (local people who want to deter amateur hunters are generally suspected); and some regulations restricting the recovery of gems are in place. Nevertheless, none of the above has prevented local jade suppliers and visitors alike from finding this rare gem.

Although some adventurers dive shore here to find jade, it's more commonly searched in the sand by sight. At the tideline, this is best accomplished, though treasure hunters are advised not to turn their back to the ocean because the currents are strong. Its color cannot always identify jade — here it comes in shades of green, blue, red, black, and brown — but with its immunity to scratching, this crystal can be verified.

4. Graves Mountain, Georgia

Graves Mountain was first mined by Tiffany & Co in the 1920s, who used the rutile to polish diamonds that it unearthed. Today, this mineral-rich mountain is available for digs by invitation only for members of the Georgia Mineral Society. However, in April and October, Graves' caretaker is opening the grounds for a three-day "rock swap & digs" to the public (There will also be a barbecue, and the whole shebang arranged by a man called Junior). The entry fee to the public event is through donations.

5. Cherokee Ruby & Sapphire Mine, N.C.

According to the Cherokee Ruby & Sapphire Mine, a rare type of stone, known as the pigeon-blood ruby, can be found here. They are more expensive than your typical stone — an extraordinarily large one was sold for $33 M at the 2015 auction — but some claim that this distinction would only apply to particular Burmese-born rubies.

Nevertheless, there are many other crystals, including good ol' natural rubies, including sapphires, moonstone, quartz, smokey quartz, and more. "Digging" is performed using soil buckets (as opposed to a search into the actual earth). However, unlike some crystal mines, Cherokee doesn't "salt" these treasure troves, which means they don't throw in gems outside to sweeten the deal for consumers. The tunnel will be closed from November through May. Fees are $25 per person.

6. Quartz Crystal Mine Wegner, Arkansas

This property is known for quartz crystals-you guessed it. And while you're not going to see anything quite that exceptional in scale, clusters are often uncovered here weighing several tons, and gems are plentiful by all accounts.

At Wegner, there are five choices to break stones. The first involves the search by sight and hand tool for a 40-acre surface mine. The second includes reaching the sluicing trough, where you can search for crystals by a pail of dirt like rubies, tourmalines, opals, amethysts, etc. The third choice is digging through a patch of dirt; which was brought down from the mine, and is periodically salted to replenish its crystal content. The fourth includes a dig at what is called the Phantom Mine, where you can find the Phantoms called rare crystals-trapped-inside-of-another-crystal. Finally, the last option involves hunting diamonds through a bag of dirt that is guaranteed to contain at least 1/2-carat of diamonds. Fees commence at $10.50 per user.